DISCIPLESHIP
5K

A Physical and Spiritual
Journey to the Cross

HEATHER NEDS

WESTBOW
PRESS®
A DIVISION OF THOMAS NELSON
& ZONDERVAN

WestBow Press books may be ordered through booksellers or by contacting:

WestBow Press
A Division of Thomas Nelson & Zondervan
1663 Liberty Drive
Bloomington, IN 47403
www.westbowpress.com
844-714-3454

ISBN: 978-1-6642-6768-8 (sc)
ISBN: 978-1-6642-6767-1 (e)

Library of Congress Control Number: 2022910075

Print information available on the last page.

WestBow Press rev. date: 06/08/2022

CONTENTS

For my fellow disciples in training

FOREWORD

by Bridget Dickason, OSB

Discipleship 5k: A Physical and Spiritual Journey to The Cross is the perfect book for those who want to become spiritually and physically fit. Heather Neds does a beautiful job of blending spiritual reflection and physical exercise in the daily reflection and physical routines she suggests. This book is a product of COVID-19. Not that the virus caused the writing of the book, but it allowed the author time to reflect and write something she has felt called to do for some time. In the spirit of Pope John XXIII's call to read the "signs of time" and Vatican II's call for the laity to reclaim their role in discipleship, Heather Neds offers readers a plan that engages mind and body, soul and flesh. She empowers them to own the discipleship to which they are called and to build spiritual and physical stamina that is required on the journey to the cross.

Discipleship in its most narrow definition was reserved for the original twelve apostles of Jesus, as seen in Matthew's gospel (Matt 10:1-15). However, even Matthew in chapter 28, verse 19 commissions the apostles to make disciples of all nations. Gospel writers Mark and Luke have a broader view of discipleship referring to 70 or 72 disciples sent forth to proclaim the Kingdom of God (Mark 3:13-19 and Luke 6:12-16). In Acts of the Apostles, all Christians of Jerusalem are called disciples (Acts 6: 1-7). Among these were women; Tabitha being the only one mentioned by name (Acts 9:36). In its broadest definition, disciple means anyone who follows the teaching of Christ or any charismatic leader.

In the 1st century, martyrdom showed one's commitment to discipleship. By the 3rd century virginity was another way to follow Christ, which gave birth to monasticism. In the 12th century, St. Francis added service to the poor as a sign of discipleship and it appeared to be restricted to religious and clergy. The Reformation and Vatican II restored discipleship to all Christians. So how do we reclaim our right to discipleship? We go back to the source of Christ's teachings in scripture. This is the first step (pun intended) of each day in this book; reflect on the Word of God and what it is calling you to do. *Lectio Divina* is an ancient form of digesting the Scripture for the spiritual journey. It feeds the soul in understanding its own salvation history through regular practice.

Anyone with some years under their belt knows that faith is a journey. Like any journey, we need to prepare. I am not a runner, but I am a seeker of God. I know life's journey is a marathon and not a sprint. I had many spiritual sprints in my youth. Those sprints led me to Benedictine monasticism in Atchison, KS. The Rule of St. Benedict's Prologue begins with "Listen, carefully, my [child], to the master's instruction, and attend to them with the ear of your heart." *Lectio Divina* is one way, or practice, of listening with the ear of our heart. The Prologue ends with, verse 49-50, "But as we advance in the monastic virtue and in faith, the heart expands, and we will run the path of God's commandments in the inexpressible delight of love. So never departing from the teachings of God, and faithfully observing His doctrine in the monastery with perseverance until death, we shall share in the sufferings of Christ, so that we may deserve also to share in His kingdom. Amen." Thousands of Benedictines and Benedictine Oblates have embraced this teaching into their own discipleship journey.

I am more of a walker and would be at Level One in Heather's book, where she breaks the marathon of faith's journey into spiritual 5K's. A 5K is the shortest long distance road running competition. It is a little over three miles. It is popular because most people can take part with no long-distance training. Health care organizations and professionals also recommend it. Regular 5K runs improve cardiovascular function and reduces body fat, as well as having mental health benefits. The 'runner's high' offers contentment and peace.

I believe Heather's blend of reflection and exercise can help the reader reach this contentment and peace. We all feel the weight of the cross in our lives at times, some more than others, making our goals feel just out of reach. How do we cope with the prolonged challenges in life? Like Christ, we are called to take up our cross and carry it daily. As each step gets harder to take, we strive to have faith that the Paschal Mystery will ring true; the cross, our personal suffering and spiritual deaths will lead to resurrection. Even Jesus had a hard time seeing it on the cross as He cried out, "my God, my God, why have you forsaken me?" (Matt 27:46), but He gave himself up to it and 'the rest is history' as they say. This book is for those who want to improve their spiritual and physical stamina at this point in their lives. It can help them process their personal salvation history on this journey we call life.

I first met Heather Neds at Keeler Women's Center in Kansas City, Kansas, when she was searching for a spiritual director in 2010. I had just finished almost twenty-five years in the high school education field and gotten my spiritual direction certification through our Souljourners Program at Mount St. Scholastica in Atchison, KS. At the time, she was Director of the Youth Ministry at Holy Family parish. I was amazed at her ability to juggle family, work, and a personal relationship with God. I was inspired to journey with this woman of faith, a true disciple, and wife, and mother, and spiritual youth leader.

The next 5K leg of Heather's life called her to deeper discipleship in the development of the Yellow Brick Foundation, an organization designed to help motivated clients overcome obstacles in their lives through long term support and education. There she developed abiding relationships with clients to assist them in building the self-esteem needed for success in achieving one's goals. During this time, she also partnered with Keeler Women's Center, starting the Scripture Study group in 2013 which she continues to lead as I write this Foreword. She attended spiritual direction, the Holy Women series, job coaching and resume writing, as well as nutrition classes. She gave back by teaching parenting classes, presenting in the Holy Women series, and offering classes on prayer and movement, homemade cleaning supplies and beauty products, and shopping the grocery ads.

Heather is preparing for the next 5K, moving from Missouri, and beginning her life in Texas. She continues to inspire me and others because of her openness to the Holy Spirit and her patience in waiting for God's direction. I look forward to seeing what God has in store for the next leg of her journey.

PREFACE

Jesus said, "Come, Follow Me" (Matt 4:19). This is easier said than done. Although I have known Jesus since I was first introduced to Him by my Great-Grandmother, Leona, I never really knew Him until I became an adult. Although raised in the Catholic Church, I stepped away for a few years at the beginning of my marriage to attend a Christian Church. I was naïve to think it wouldn't matter where I worshiped.

It did matter and I realized it while I was sitting in the congregation on the day of my second daughter's dedication in the Christian Church. I missed the sacred connection and ritual I'd grown up with through the sacraments. I wanted to connect with God on a deeper level and that wasn't going to happen at the church where I was attending.

The journey to a deeper relationship led me to recommitting myself to the Catholic faith. I attended a retreat where I was reminded how special the sacraments are, not only in the Catholic Church but how special they had come to be for me in my life. I left the retreat with a fire within me and a rededication to who I was in Christ and for Christ.

I knew I wanted to have a relationship with Jesus and if it was going to be any good, I would need to dedicate more time and attention to cultivating that relationship. The Pastor at my church saw my desire to learn and thought my newfound passion to grow in faith would be a good example for the youth. I found myself teaching and leading high school teens at the church and within six months, I was asked to work with the teens on a full-time basis.

In my 15 years as a youth minister, I attended several workshops and conferences where I gathered and learned more about being a disciple of Jesus. However, a problem existed. I was spending time consuming information and found myself confusing the time I was studying about faith and spirituality as spending time with God and building my relationship with Him.

My turning point, like many, was during a time when I felt despair and turned to God for help. I will never forget the day when I was lying face-down on the carpet below the crucifix at the church sobbing. As I lay prostrate at the foot of the cross, I surrendered my life to Christ and promised to put more effort into growing my faith and relationship with Jesus. My promise meant I would need to do things differently.

I was reminded of a keynote I had heard titled, *Faith Horticulturist*, by my friend, Catholic speaker, Mike Patin. He said Jesus used three basic tools to plant the seeds of faith in His followers: the Bible, a towel, and the Cross. I figured if they are good enough for Jesus to use, then they are good enough for me. I started to study Scripture more diligently and looked for opportunities to be of service to others.

It didn't take long for me to see I still had a roadblock in my way. In the Scripture passage when Jesus was asked about which of the commandments was the most important; "He said to love God with all your heart, mind, and spirit; and to love others as yourself" (Matt 22:34-40, author's paraphrase). I realized if I was going to be working on loving God better, I also needed to love myself better. This meant I needed to be able to look in the mirror and be proud of who I am. I needed to love myself.

For years, I measured my self-worth by what I looked like and how much I weighed. As far back as middle school, I practiced aerobic exercise and tried new diet after new diet to manage weight. I was not going to be held back by my own self-image and knew I needed to begin making it a priority to live a healthier lifestyle. This meant making time for myself to exercise and to begin to make better choices when eating. I wanted to change my habits and then it occurred to me that I can combine my reflection and study time with my workout time.

In the past I had made excuses for not spending time with God, just like I did for not taking care of my body physically. It was time for me to stop making excuses. I needed my lifestyle to reflect what I said I believed so if I said my relationship with God was important and I wanted to live a healthy lifestyle, then I needed to start doing it.

This time starting a new exercise regimen was combined with my time in prayer. I had a new, not so secret weapon on my side, Jesus, to push me through. I did not want to let Him down, so I turned to the Scripture when Jesus called the first disciples to begin my journey. I knew the scripture already, but when I read it this time, I felt an immediate connection to it, as though I too was being called to follow Him.

Jesus did not tell the disciples the journey would be easy, He only asked them to leave their nets behind and follow. If He had given them the job description, telling them it would require sacrifice, demanding work, and endurance to follow Him, perhaps they would have remained there by the seashore. I took to heart that to be a disciple of Jesus, one needs to have discipline and I believe it is not a coincidence that you cannot spell discipline without disciple!

It is because of the success I found combining my physical and spiritual journey that the *Discipleship 5K* came to fruition. I found strength in the Scripture to help push me through a tough workout routine. I reached out to others for encouragement and gave it back to them. I battled the negative forces, externally and internally, and came out victorious because God was there by my side. And through the process, I believe God gifted me with more time to be of service to others and called me to help lead them to the cross.

This book is designed to be a guide. I wrote it with the expectation that each person will approach it at their own pace. Some who begin the challenge may not be physically active and the physical piece may sound overwhelming, so they will want to take it slowly, or omit the physical piece altogether. There is no right or wrong way to put the physical and spiritual exercises into practice in your life. It is meant to be a tool to help give support and direction towards the goal of being a better disciple.

Although, I find it imperative for everyone who begins this challenge to know that it can change your life. As I spent time in prayer, reflection, and service, I learned things about myself and others that caused me to make different decisions about how and with whom I spent my time. I found as my body changed, I was more energetic and wanted to be more active. I came to appreciate the simple things and lived more in the present, seeing life as it is right now and not as something it was in the past or how I want it to be in the future.

Just as it is said, you cannot judge a book by its cover, I believe you cannot judge a person from their exterior either. "God said He created man and woman in His image, but the likeness is not what is on the outside; it is on the inside where God dwells" (Gen 1:26-27, author's paraphrase). There is more than meets the eye in each person you meet, including yourself. On my journey I learned to see myself as God sees me, fearfully and wonderfully made (Ps 139:14). This perspective gave me a new awareness not only of myself but of others as well.

Yes, the title of the book is the *Discipleship 5K*, but the main focus is not for you to enter an actual 5K race, though it is certainly a carrot you can use to motivate yourself to continue to move forward. You are already a part of the human race; the race of life and this book will help you prepare to be the disciple you were born to be. These pages will help you identify your God given gifts and challenge you to see yourself as God sees you, as a disciple of Jesus.

If you accept this challenge, you will discover new things about yourself and see others in a different way too. You will not only be able to see a change in your body as it becomes stronger and more agile, but you will have a brighter more positive outlook about life in general. This challenge requires you to work on the outside, the physical but also the inside, the spiritual, to find out what you are made of, and I imagine you have barely scratched the surface of what you can achieve.

ACKNOWLEDGEMENTS

First, I acknowledge God for calling me into being and planting within me the desire to teach. As a little girl, I remember setting all my stuffed animals on my bed as though they were students and playing school. I also loved to look at and read the stories of my Children's Bible. These two things, teaching and learning about God have been at the center of my life, leading me to where I am today. Along the way, I have shared all I have learned about faith with my family as a wife and mother, as a youth minister. I shared my love for Jesus in a church, as a substitute teacher in Catholic schools, and continued to live out my faith as the co-founder of The Yellow Brick Foundation, a nonprofit organization, and of course by leading Bible studies. I believe this is my purpose in life and am grateful God continues to give me opportunities to share His Word with others.

I give thanks to all my teachers, those who have taught me about faith. Thank you to my first teachers, my parents, my grandparents, and great-grandparents, as well as extended family members who first introduced me to Jesus and God's unconditional love.

Thank you to the saints who shared their stories and inspired me, specifically, Saint Teresa of Avila, Saint Teresa of Calcutta, Saint Gianna Beretta Molla, Saint Augustine, and Pope John Paul II.

Thank you to the religious leaders in my life including Father Robert, Father Matthew, Father Bob, Father Ken, Father Paul, Father Don, Father Joe, Monsignor Brad, Bishop Boland, and Bishop Finn, all of whom affected my personal and professional life and taught me valuable faith lessons.

Thank you to faith leaders, J. Glenn Murray, Father James Martin, Thomas Merton, Richard Rohr, David Hass, Robert Wicks, Mary McKenna, Matthew Kelly, Andy Andrews, and countless others whose words have infected me, causing me to wrestle with who I am, what I believe and why I believe it. I am grateful to all the keynote speakers and workshop presenters who shared their insight and expertise at the many conferences and retreats I have attended. I continue to learn and grow in my faith because of the wisdom you share.

Thank you to my faith friends, especially Elizabeth and Mike, both of whom have supported my learning and growing in faith. For over 20 years they have been walking alongside me, encouraging, and challenging me to step outside my comfort zone or to go the extra mile. Also, to the many friends and colleagues with whom I have shared time with on retreat or attended conferences. The time we shared together in prayer and the conversations about faith, life, and God is where I am able to mold and shape my values and become clear about my beliefs. There have been many over the years but each of you has played a role in my faith development. You have a special place in my heart, and I am so glad our paths crossed and perhaps will again one day.

I also give thanks to my Bible study ladies and all those at Keeler Women's Center, especially Sister Carol Ann, Sister Bridget, Sister Patricia, Sister Barbara, Brenda, Carolyn, Pat, Joanna, Arnita, Eartha, Lisa, Patricia, Heather, Diane, Susie, and others who joined us for a season or two. Thank you for allowing me to share faith with you and for sharing your faith with me. I reflect often on our discussions and much of what is in this book comes from our time reflecting on the Scripture together. Also, thank you so much for encouraging me to put my scripture studies out into the world to share. You all have contributed to this work and my development of being a better disciple.

Thank you to my editors, Barb, Peggy, and Judy. I am grateful for you, for your support and your input on this project. I cannot put into words how much I appreciate the time and effort you shared and the accountability you gave me to complete it.

Thank you, Jane Fonda, Suzanne Summers, Gilad, Denise

Austin, Richard Simmons, Brooke Burke, and all the fitness video kings and queens I grew up knowing. As early as middle school I was a consumer of these videos and physical fitness routines. Over the years, I have learned so much from the instructors of Pilates, Yoga, Zumba and HIIT classes I have attended, each helping me to feel strong and confident, even when I could not do the exercise or pose correctly. They helped me become comfortable in my own skin and accept my limitations, as well as learn to laugh at myself. I am also glad I read Tom Brady's book about the TB12 Method because it solidified for me the importance of taking care of my body so I can be physically able to do the things I want to be able to do in my life.

Finally, thank you to my daughters, Courtney, AnnaLee and Madison, whose lives have blessed mine so deeply. Becoming a mom, is one of my favorite gifts from God. They enlighten me and delight me with their beauty inside and out. And thank you to my husband Ron who has been one of my greatest examples of God's love, grace, mercy, and forgiveness. God gave me the right partner to do life with, one who supports me and brings out the best in me. Thank you.

INTRODUCTION

Before you begin, there are a few things you might consider getting or having on hand to help set you up for success. Just as you would pack a bag for an overnight or weekend trip with items that would be considered essential such as your toothbrush, toothpaste, or your underwear there are some things that could make this journey a bit smoother.

It is highly recommended, if you do not have a good pair of walking or running shoes as well as good socks, you should plan to purchase these items. Appropriate clothing is needed whether you are training indoors or outdoors. If you are new to physical activity, it might take a little time to determine what type of clothing is the most comfortable for you. It is not necessary for you to get a gym membership or buy any special gear unless you feel it will keep you motivated. Sometimes when you invest money into a project, you become more inclined to follow through with it because you want to get your money's worth. Joining a gym could also provide you with an accountability piece because you could join a class where people will miss you if you are not there.

You will also need a way to keep track of your mileage and rate of movement. There are several free apps for smart phones or other devices that you can get to track your movement. You could also choose to use one of several wrist bands or smart watches to help measure your speed and distance. The key is to pick something that is convenient and easy for you to use because you do not want it to become a stress in your life.

For the spiritual training, you will use this book as a journal to help keep track of your thoughts. You will also need to have a Bible to look up the scripture for each day. It is encouraged that you look up the scripture and read it a few times to prayerfully listen to what

God wants you to hear. Reading the scripture aloud is also highly recommended.

The intended practice for your spiritual training is formally called *Lectio Divina,* which is an ancient form of prayer. Basically, it means each day you will read the daily scripture to yourself, then sit in silence, allowing the Word to penetrate your body. After a minute or so, prayerfully read the same verse aloud. This means slowly and with purpose. Then read the scripture passage again and sit in silence, this time allowing the scripture to sift through your brain until a word or phrase stands out. These words can sometimes point out a solution to a problem, stir up a memory, and sometimes present new insights into your personal or professional life. Before you get started, it would be good to grab a composition book, a notebook, or a journal to keep on hand in case you find you want added space to write out your thoughts.

Additionally, there are several spiritual resources you can gain access to online or through an app. These are helpful for daily inspiration and easy access for spiritual reading whenever you find yourself with a few spare minutes of time. You can also find and follow people and organizations on social media platforms. Many of these daily reflections are free and can come to you through your email or in your social media feed, which makes it easy and convenient to connect to God's Word.

If you would like resources specific to *Discipleship 5K,* it is recommended you find and follow the *Making Scripture Relevant* page on Facebook and/or Instagram. There you can get daily prayers and reflections written by the author, Heather Neds. On the Facebook page, there is a group specifically for *Discipleship 5K* participants to have discussions, ask questions, and give/receive affirmations with others reading the book. Joining this group is optional but it is a wonderful way to be connected to others on the same *Discipleship 5K* journey. There are also daily videos on the *Making Scripture Relevant* YouTube channel where you can watch Heather Neds discuss the scripture, shares ideas, and give motivation to participants. These resources were created to help you stay on course and support you along the way.

As you set out, remember you are not in this race alone because disciples are called out to travel together. The Bible says Jesus sent His disciples out two by two (Mark 6:7), so even if you choose to go through the book alone, there are others out there ready and willing to offer support and encouragement. Plus, there are times during the journey when you will be asked to reach out to others and encourage them or to ask them to join you for a walk or to attend a cardio or yoga class together; this is primarily to remind you that disciples need one another for support and accountability.

Lastly, you might consider joining forces with a group and meeting each week to check in with one another on the highs and lows of your experience. You could coordinate a new group at your church or community center or suggest an existing group to use *Discipleship 5K* as their next bible study or book club book. You can also use the book as a family, adapting one of the spiritual practices suggested for each week to do together and making time to participate in some sort of physical activity together. Regardless of how you decide to take part in the *Discipleship 5K*, the important part is that you are setting yourself up with the resources you need to stay on course and have fun along the way.

DESCRIPTION OF ACTIVITIES

PHYSICAL TRAINING

Each person needs to figure out a personal goal based on their physical abilities. Throughout the book there will be suggested physical activities given to help you train for a race. These are only suggestions and will vary depending on each person's physical abilities and their personal goals. There will be suggestions for three different activity levels.

> Level 1: for someone whose physical activity is at a minimum or just beginning
> Level 2: for someone who is moderately active and leads a semi-active lifestyle
> Level 3: for someone who regularly exercise and aspires to literally go the distance

Feel free to mix and match these levels, stick to just one or even make up your own. You know your body best, so listen to it and acknowledge your limitations. If you push yourself too hard, you risk injury and that will increase your likelihood of quitting. You also know when you need to take a rest or when you have a little extra to give. The ACTION suggested for each day is simply that, a suggestion.

CROSS-TRAINING ACTIVITY

These activities include cycling indoors or outdoors at a light to moderate pace to get your heart rate up; swimming laps, also at a light to moderate pace enough for your heart rate to go up; or attending a cardio class such as Zumba, aerobics, or kickboxing. You can find free apps with cross-training activities or find a community center where you can attend classes, usually for a minimal fee.

The purpose of cross-training is to build and strengthen muscles that you do not use when you are walking or running. You do not want to over work those muscles, but you also do not want to slow down your momentum of staying regularly active. Participating in a cross-training activity will give the muscles you do regularly use a break and strengthen other muscles that provide support to those muscles. All your muscles are connected, and these other activities supply opportunity to work on your entire body, not just one specific area. It is also important that you get your heart rate up when you do your cross-training activity so you can build up your endurance and strengthen your heart.

WEIGHT TRAINING ACTIVITY

You can lift free weights, use a machine, or even use household items to build up strength. If you do not have a weight machine or free weights at home, you can grab a couple of cand from your pantry, a sack of sugar or your laundry detergent to complete your training regimen for the day. Lifting weights can help build muscles to protect your bones. It is not necessary to lift heavy weights, rather it is recommended you use smaller weights with more repetition. The purpose of this is to help build endurance by strengthening the muscles.

The focus of weight training as part of *Discipleship 5K* is not the amount of weight you lift, instead it is the practice of a discipline. As with cross-training, you lift weights to build and strengthen muscles you do not use while walking or running so your entire body becomes stronger. If you do not have experience with weight training, there are several videos and apps with pointers on proper techniques to avoid injury.

YOGA AND STRETCHING

This can be done on your own, using an app, or by attending a class at a studio, gym, or community center. You could even purchase a book of basic stretches or borrow one from the library to get ideas of how to stretch different parts of your body. The purpose of practicing yoga and deep stretching is to help prevent injury. You achieve this by not only stretching the muscles and ligaments but also strengthening the little muscles surrounding the bigger muscles used when walking or running.

If you are just beginning, do not expect to be able to do all the poses suggested by an instructor. You must honor the limitations of your body and be gentle with yourself. Through regular practice you may find your body becoming more limber so do not get discouraged, just do your best.

Throughout the book, you will be reminded to stretch. This is because stretching helps prevent injury, and it can minimize cramps or soreness following a workout. It is one of those things that is easy to skip, but it is an important part of the process, so make the time to do it.

This step is also important because it gives you the opportunity to stop and focus on your body. When you stretch, you may feel tightness in a specific area of your body, which is a clue that you might need to take it easy. So be sure to stretch before and after your scheduled exercise every day.

CALISTHENICS

These are the classic sit-ups, push-ups, jumping jacks, and lunges everyone loved to hate in gym class. As with the previous activities, the purpose of doing calisthenics is to build and strengthen your muscles so when called upon to do something hard, you have the endurance to persevere. There are apps you can use to guide you through a variety of exercises to do or create your own routine. Just like with yoga and deep stretching, you need to listen to your body and honor its limitations. For example, if you have knee problems, it is probably best for you not to do jumping jacks. When choosing the type of activities you will do, be smart.

DEEP BREATHING

It may sound silly to encourage you to breathe, but it is an important piece to both the physical and spiritual part of the *Discipleship 5K* journey. Breathing is something you do naturally, without thinking, but when you pay attention to your breath, you can learn to use it to do so much more than just keep you alive. When you pay attention to your breathing it can help your body perform at its best. Integrating several types of breaths or breathing techniques such as pushing air in and out through your nose or your mouth; or breathing into your belly or into your chest can increase your capacity, thus improve performance.

You will be encouraged to practice your breathing throughout *Discipleship 5K*. You can find out more about the different ways to breathe and the benefits of deep breathing or meditation online, in an app, or from a research book. There are also several podcasts where they discuss the benefits and specific techniques to practice the different types of breathing.

The goal is for you to find a breathing practice that works best for you. Learning how to breath in different ways can help you both physically and spiritually. It will help you physically by building the capacity of your lungs so when you walk or run, you will not lose your breath right away. The greatest benefit spiritually is becoming mindful of God's presence in your breath. After all, it was God who breathed life into you in the first place, what better way is there to connect with God!

DISTANCE

Whether your goal is to take part in a 5K race or not, it is good to know how many miles it is; 3.1 miles. The very first day you begin *Discipleship 5K*, your first task is to set your goal in time and distance. You many set a goal of being able to walk three miles in an hour or you may want to be able to run the same three miles in 30 minutes.

The most popular race distances are:

5K = 3.1 miles
10K = 6.2 miles
½ Marathon = 13.1 miles
Full Marathon = 26.2 miles

Discipleship 5K: A Physical and Spiritual Journey to the Cross is not an exercise program and does not guarantee weight loss. When you participate in any physical activity, you risk the chance of injury. Be sure to consult your physician to ensure you are physically able to take part in the activities suggested.

WEEK ONE
Get Ready to Begin

It is important to work on your body, mind, and spirit to support wellness. *Discipleship 5K* is a framework created to help you work on all three. Start your exercise time with prayer by reading the daily scripture, the reflection, and journal exercise. Then as you work on your physical fitness, you will spend the time thinking about what you just read, allowing God's Word to motivate you to do your best. Your workout time will become sacred time because you will be meditating on God's Word and reflecting on how you will complete the journal exercise. Throughout the *Discipleship 5K* you will be building your muscles to make you physically stronger, but you will also grow spiritually by connecting daily to scripture and deepening your relationship with God and with others. It is time to begin.

DAY 1

Set Goals

Scripture: 1 Timothy 4:6-15

> Train yourself in godliness, for, while physical training is of some value, godliness is valuable in every way, holding promise for both the present life and the life to come. (1 Tim 4:7b-8)

REFLECTION

These words from Saint Paul to Timothy were written to encourage Timothy so he would not get discouraged. Saint Paul wanted to get Timothy excited about the challenge ahead of him of training new Christians on how to live as disciples. Discipleship takes intention and hard work. This scripture passage is the perfect starting point as you take on the challenge of building a stronger relationship with God while tackling physical challenges. There will be times when you, like Timothy, will need a pep talk to stay motivated.

If you want to be a better disciple, then you must train. Athletes, musicians, scientists, teachers, electricians, and anyone who wants to be better at their job, train and practice. Training helps you gain the skills you need to do your job well and the repetitiveness of practice gives you the opportunity to sharpen those skills to the point where you complete the task fluidly. You have been given the gift of faith and in the words of Saint Paul in the Scripture, it is time to "put it into practice, devote yourself to it, so you can see your progress" (1 Tim 4:15).

JOURNAL

As you get started, it is good to map out your physical goals and your spiritual goals. Look at these goals often to help you stay focused on what you wish to achieve. Let them serve as a guide to keep you motivated to work towards being a stronger you both physically and spiritually. Your soul-training starts now.

Write down the physical goals you want to work towards and be specific.

> What do you want to achieve by the end of the challenge physically?

> Do you want to increase the amount of time you spend doing intentional exercise?

> Do you want to walk or run a 5K?

> Do you want to be able to play catch with your kids and not feel winded?

> Do you want to lose weight?

> Do you have a specific distance you wish to reach?

Write down any other thoughts you have about your physical journey.

Write down the spiritual goals you want to work towards and be specific.

> Do you want to deepen your relationship with God?

Do you want to be more like Jesus? In what way(s)?

Do you want your faith to be the first thing people see when they meet you?

Do you want to know yourself better?

Do you want to pray more regularly?

Do you want to read more scripture?

Write down any other thoughts about your spiritual journey.

ACTION

Though this is called *Discipleship 5K*, you do not need to walk or run a 5K. This challenge is open for you to set personal goals to fit your own physical ability. Throughout the book, the reference to the 5K is a general term to stand for your physical goal.

> Level 1: walk as long and as far as you can to find your starting point. If it is for 5 minutes or 50 minutes this will help you decide at which rate to continue from and then plan to build on this distance and/or time
> Level 2: walk 3.1 miles (5K) and note your time
> Level 3: run 3.1 miles (5K) and note your time

What is your time today?   What is your distance today?
What is your goal time?   What is your goal distance?

DAY 2

Identify Obstacles

Scripture: Genesis 32:24-30

> Jacob said, "I will not let you go, unless you bless me." (Gen 32:26b)

REFLECTION

Today's scripture is a story about Jacob wrestling with God. There may be days when you feel like Jacob as you work through this book. You might even wrestle with God as you face physical and spiritual challenges. There will be obstacles that keep you from doing the daily work suggested in *Discipleship 5K* and you might beat yourself up about missing a day or not giving an exercise or prayer your all. It is bound to happen whenever you start on a new path because your old ways are more comfortable. However, God does not call disciples to do easy things. A disciple must face challenges, overcome obstacles, and sometimes even suffer pain.

Jacob wrestles with God all night and when the morning comes, he asks God to give him His blessing. Why would Jacob want God to bless him, after he struck his hip out of joint? Perhaps it is a reminder that there will be some hard days ahead. The struggle did not scare Jacob away from moving forward and it should not stop you either. Jacob's experience is an example for you to remain focused on your goal even through the tough times because God is there with you and will help you prevail.

At the end of the scripture passage, God does give Jacob the blessing he asked for, but He also changed Jacob's name to Israel. When this happens in Scripture, for example Abram to Abraham and Simon to Peter, it is a sign of conversion. The blessing is God saying, you are His chosen one and He expects you to step up with all you have, to take on the task in front of you. God had big plans for Jacob, but He also has big plans for you. This is important to remember as you do the physical and spiritual work each day.

Discipleship 5K is an opportunity to mold and shape your character. God puts challenges in your path so you can learn something along the way. If you skim over or skip out of an experience, then you might miss out on a lesson God wants you to learn to build your character. Your experiences and how you deal with problems will help you become a better disciple. Are you ready to begin your wrestling match with God?

JOURNAL

Take time to name things that could cause you to stumble or fall during this challenge. When you name the obstacles, you can be ready for battle when you come face to face with them. Set yourself up for success by writing down anything that could get in your way of doing your best. It could be something such as a sore muscle, it is too hard, you cannot find the time or a thousand other things. Make a list of potential obstacles for the physical side of the challenge and also for the spiritual side, even if some of the obstacles you list are the same for each side. Be as specific as you can so when they come up you can prevail like Jacob did when wrestling with God.

> List potential obstacles that could come up and
> keep you from taking part in the physical activities.

List potential obstacles that could come up and keep you from taking part in the spiritual activities.

ACTION

Be sure to use your whole body as you breathe, paying attention to the expansion of your belly as your body fills with air and then the emptiness you feel as you push every bit of it out. Practice breathing deeply for at least 5 minutes.

Level 1: no physical exercise but practice breathing deeply
Level 2: do 15-20 minutes of yoga or stretching
Level 3: do 30-60 minutes of yoga or stretching

DAY 3

Choose Holiness

Scripture: Leviticus 19-20

> You shall be holy, for I the Lord your God am holy.
> (Lev 19:2)

REFLECTION

Today's agenda includes reading chapters 19 & 20 in the book of Leviticus. God tells the Israelites to be holy as He is holy. It is equivalent to the Ten Commandments where God lays down the law, telling them what they can do (Lev 19) and cannot do (Lev 20). They needed guidance, guidelines to help them. People, since Adam and Eve have needed help staying out of trouble. So, when you lose your way and get off track, it is only natural. People have been having a tough time determining the difference between right and wrong since the beginning of time. The Scripture gives detailed instructions of what to do and what not to do. This is helpful.

The purpose of *Discipleship 5K* is to help you become more disciplined and be holy as God is holy. When you wake up each morning, you have a choice whether it is going to be a good day or a not so good day before you even get out of bed by seeking God first. When you ask God to guide your day and to help you make good choices, you are more likely to have a good day. The Israelites in the scripture struggled with relying on God to help them with their everyday activities. Turn to God first and ask Him to help you make good choices so at the end of the day, even if you faced some challenges, you will be able to say you had a good day. This is the kind of work you need to do to be a better disciple.

JOURNAL

It is self-reflection time. As you move your body physically, contemplate these questions, then write down your answers. This will help you stay accountable to the changes you wish to make throughout the process. Answer these questions honestly as it truly is and not how you want it to be.

How do you treat your friends?

How do you spend your money?

How much time do you spend alone with God?

Does the music you listen to reflect your relationship with God?

Do the TV shows and movies you watch reflect your relationship with God?

If a stranger looked at your social media feeds, would they know you had a relationship with God?

How do you reflect holiness in your life?

Spend time meditating and praying about the answers.
Write down a one sentence mantra to help you to
choose God to be a part of your everyday life.

ACTION

Spend at least 5 minutes practicing your breathing by taking deep breaths in through your nose and filling your stomach with air. If it helps, put your hands on your stomach to feel the expansion.

Level 1: do 10-15 minutes of yoga or stretching and
remember to breathe during the practice
Level 2: do 20-30 minutes of a cross-training activity
Level 3: do 60-90 minutes of a cross-training activity

DAY 4

Let Go

Scripture: Ecclesiastes 11:7-10

> Banish anxiety from your mind and put away pain
> from your body. (Eccl 11:10a)

REFLECTION

When you were young, you probably took more chances and did not weigh out the consequences of your actions the way you do now. Young people do not reflect on life the way older people do, they simply go out and live it. Thankfully, youthfulness is a state of mind which you can cultivate even when you are older.

Do not allow yourself to sit on the sidelines of life because of anxiety or pain. You have the choice to either give up, allowing these obstacles to put you on the bench or to find ways to overcome the obstacles so you can get in the game. The tools described in *Discipleship 5K* can help give you permission to pause and reflect on your life and how you live it. These reflections can reveal new perspectives and possibilities you might not have considered before. Embrace the obstacles so you can grow into the disciple you want to be.

Jesus said, "Truly I tell you, unless you change and become like children, you will never enter the kingdom of heaven" (Matt 18:3). He wants you to be young at heart and the scripture verse, Ecclesiastes 11:9 confirms it by stating, "Follow the inclination of your heart." This advice to follow your heart is good advice for everyone at any age, because your heart highlights what you love and desire the most.

Today is about being reminded to listen to your heartbeat and to be grateful for each breath. The action today reflects this theme too because the goal is to push yourself a little bit to get your heart beating and lose your breath. The purpose is to remind you that you are alive. It is amazing how you do not even have to tell your heart to beat or to remind yourself to take a breath, and these are the two things you need to do to stay alive.

The scripture says each day you live, your purpose is to love God and to be loved by God. Throughout your life there will be things that weigh you down and cause you stress or anxiety. When you focus on loving God and allowing God to love you, the things that seem to overwhelm you can begin to look more manageable. The practice of meditation is a terrific way to release stress and a wonderful way to be reminded of God's love by paying attention to your breath and heartbeat.

JOURNAL

Spend 5-10 minutes in silence today listening to your heartbeat. While you sit listening to your heart, see if you can hear what your heart is saying to you. Today is a gift from God and He's waiting to spend time with you.

> Write down what you hear your heartbeat tell you. (For example, does it tell you that you worry too much? You put too much stress on it? Do you hear it tell you about your dreams and where it wants to lead you?)

Write down the things that cause you stress.

How do these things affect your physical health?

How do these things affect your spiritual health?

What are the benefits of letting go of these things and focusing on the goals you have set?

ACTION

Rev up the physical action today by pushing yourself a little bit so you can catch your breath and feel your heart pumping. Do not skimp on the stretching as it is a perfect time to breathe deeply and connect with God. For an extra challenge, see if you can take a step with each beat of your heart.

Level 1: walk ¼ or ½ a mile as fast as you can and do 5 minutes of calisthenics before and after your walk
Level 2: run 1-2 miles at your peak pace and do 10 minutes of calisthenics before and after your run
Level 3: run 2-5 miles at your peak pace and do 10 minutes of calisthenics before and after your run

DAY 5

Find Encouragement

Scripture: Philippians 1:3-11

> I am confident of this, that the one who began a good
> work among you will bring it to completion. (Phil 1:6)

REFLECTION

"You've got a friend in me" is a Randy Newman song from the
movie *Toy Story* and it is the perfect theme song for today. Saint Paul
is sending words of encouragement to his friends in the scripture
passage, letting them know that those who have begun practicing
the disciplines of being a Christian will achieve their goal. He
encourages the Philippians to stay on course despite the difficulties
of their everyday lives. He is saying there will be challenges along
the way, but one step back does not mean you are done. Saint
Paul's words are designed to encourage you too. They are a perfect
reminder as you begin this challenge. You know you will experience
difficulties as you try new exercises and spend more time focused
on your faith life, but you are doing a good thing for your body and
your spirit, so keep up the excellent work.

Most people first learn that Jesus is your friend. Maybe you sang
the song, "You've got a friend in Jesus" as a child at church. This initial
introduction to Jesus was to show the human side of God. It is through
Jesus that you learn about true friendship, how you should care for
one another and want the best for them. Jesus teaches this in the Bible
when He shows compassion through healing the sick and the lame,
and He models acceptance of all people through acts of service. Jesus
shared parables, modern day stories to teach everyone how to live out
the commandments, and specifically how to love God and love others.

It is important to understand that the people you surround yourself with affects your attitude and behavior. When you surround yourself with a community of people who have common goals, you can celebrate victories and inspire one another to do better. Be sure you are being supported by others who have shared beliefs and values and/or help you find the things you deem most important. It is through the support of others, your companions on the journey, that you will receive encouragement when you are feeling down and need to stay motivated. If you do not have people like this is your life right now, go out and find people who will love you the way God loves you.

JOURNAL

The focus today is to examine your friendships. Reflect on your friendships and if the people whom you surround yourself with encourage you and if you encourage them. It takes intention to connect with another person in a true and unselfish way. Check in to be sure the people with whom you spend the most time build you up instead of tear you down. Remember to thank Jesus for being such a wonderful role model of true friendship in your prayers today.

Make a list of people whom you call friend.

Make a list of people with whom you spend the most time.

Are the two lists above the same or different?

What are the characteristics you look for in a faithful friend?

Who do you go to when you need encouragement?

Who are the people that come to you for encouragement?

How can you put or keep Christ at the center of your friendships?

ACTION

Today while you do your action, think about those with whom you spend the most time, how you treat one another and if God is in those relationships.

Level 1: do 10-15 minutes of yoga or stretching and practicing your breathing while you stretch

Level 2: do 20-30 minutes of a cross-training activity
and spend 5 minutes practicing deep breathing
Level 3: do 60-90 minutes of a cross-training activity
and spend 5 minutes practicing deep breathing

DAY 6

Open Your Heart - Mind - Soul

Scripture: Mark 1:16-20

> And immediately they left their nets and followed
> him. (Mark 1:18)

REFLECTION

Jesus is calling the first disciples to come and follow him in the
scripture today. Jesus is calling you by name too. He calls you to
share in His mission.

It can be hard to grasp the mission you are called to be a part
of because God does not reveal the whole plan. When you do not
know what lies ahead, it can be difficult to have a cheerful outlook,
especially when it feels as if each day runs into the next. There is
hardly time to remember the choices you make and how your choices
either move you closer or farther away from God's mission.

In school, the teachers give the students a syllabus that lays out what
you will learn throughout the year and shows you how you will arrive at
the goal. Then there is a comprehensive final at the end of the class to tell
you if you passed or failed. However, how many of the students actually
look at the syllabus after that first day anyways and does knowing what
they are going to learn help them arrive at the goal any faster?

God, like the teachers in school, did give you a syllabus for life
it is called the Bible. In it, you learn about God's people, people like
you who have followed God and turned their backs on God, plus
you read about God's Law. Although you do not know the exact
path God has planned for your life, you do know that you have been
called to follow Him and that means following His commandments.
And how well you follow them is what will be on life's comprehensive

final, so your mission is to follow Jesus and open your heart, mind, and soul to Him and be His disciple at all times.

JOURNAL

The first mission is to love God with all your heart, mind, and soul. Reflect on how you do this. Take time to write down specific steps you need to take to connect to God more deeply.

What keeps you from opening yourself up completely to God?

What do you need to open your heart, mind, and soul for God?

Identify three action steps you can take to open your heart and body in this challenge.

Identify three action steps you can take to open your mind/thoughts in this challenge.

Identify three action steps you can take to open your soul/spirit in this challenge.

ACTION

You are called to love God with your heart, mind, and spirit. As you move your body, reflect on how you can do this more fully. Remember to stretch before and after your walk or jog.

Level 1: take a 1–2-mile leisurely walk
Level 2: take a 3–5-mile leisurely walk
Level 3: take a 3–5-mile leisurely jog

DAY 7

Stand Up

Scripture: Luke 9:1-6

> He sent them out to proclaim the kingdom of God.
> (Luke 9:2)

REFLECTION

The scripture today is from the Gospel of Luke when Jesus sends the disciples out to preach the gospel message. You are also called to preach the Gospel too, through your words and actions. This is not easy, because it means following God's Law which can contradict what the world says you should do. It is easier to blend in, follow popular opinion, and not be judged by others for going against the grain.

As you do the spiritual work to become a better disciple, there will be times when the mission God calls you to seems impossible. You might lose friends. You might lose your job. Therefore, it is important for you to decide now, while it is still early in the challenge, what you are willing to stand up for and if God is a part of it. Are you willing to make choices which do not follow the popular opinion because it is the right thing to do?

When asked to share in Jesus' mission, you are being asked to not follow the crowd but to follow Jesus. It is possible, but it can certainly look and feel like the odds are against you. Allow your faith to shine through as your guide, to help you reflect God's love, grace, compassion, and mercy. And on the days when it gets rough, remember you are not alone when you walk the walk and talk the talk, there are disciples everywhere, ready to stand up with you.

JOURNAL

Disciples make mistakes. Although, the more you practice doing what is right or just, even if it is in your head, the next time you are in a situation, you are more likely to have the tools you need to stand up for what you believe. If you take God along with you, you will not fail!

How often do you go along with something you do not want to do, or you know is wrong only to satisfy another person? Write about a time when you went along with a plan even though it went against what you believed to be right or just.

Imagine the scenario you described where instead of going along, you stood up for what you believe. Describe what changes in the situation, such as what is said and if the outcome is different.

Discipleship 5K

ACTION

Look back on the progress you have made this week both physically and spiritually. Practice your breathing while you stretch or do yoga.

> Level 1: take a day of rest but spend a few minutes practicing your breathing by slowly taking deep breaths in and out through your nose
> Level 2: do 15-20 minutes of yoga or stretching.
> Level 3: do 30-60 minutes of yoga or stretching.

WEEK ONE OVERVIEW

Write down any thoughts, words of encouragement, ideas for growth or measurements of progress you have from this week from your physical and spiritual training.

WEEK TWO
Tools for the Physical Journey

The physical activities in *Discipleship 5K* require you to move your body with intention. No matter what level you are at physically, there is one thing you absolutely need to be a successful walker, jogger, or runner and that is a good pair of walking or running shoes. When you do not have good shoes, you are likely to get a blister, stub a toe, or twist an ankle. You do not have to buy a new pair, but you do need to have shoes with stability and tread as you will be putting some miles on your shoes.

However, do not allow money to become an obstacle in this challenge. Your success depends on you, not the fancy shoes, socks, clothes, or workout accessories the world tells you are necessary. Instead, use what you already have in your closet, garage, or pantry. For example, if you do not have dumbbells for strength training, use canned goods or a bottle of water or some other household item for weights. Remember, the goal is to get your body moving, do not think you need to spend a bunch of money to do this challenge. Be creative and do what is comfortable for you.

Think Differently

Scripture: Genesis 27:1-40

> Cursed be everyone who curses you and blessed be
> everyone who blesses you! (Gen 27:29c)

REFLECTION

From the beginning of time, God shows up in the scripture, going against the law of the people. God's ways are different than the ways of the world. He chooses people who seem to be the least likely to be able to complete a task and He uses them to accomplish remarkable things. Think about all the people in Scripture who God chose, like David, the young shepherd boy to be king or Moses, the man with a speech impediment to lead the Israelites or even the unmarried pregnant teenager, Mary to be the mother of God's only Son, Jesus. God has a trend of taking someone the world says is unworthy or undesirable and accomplishing something great in their lives.

Perhaps this is what God is doing with you on this challenge. Maybe now after a week you are thinking you are not cut out for this physical activity. Your muscles might be sore, and possibly feeling like you took on more than you should because you just do not have the time or energy to complete the daily tasks. As a disciple, you need to think differently, you need to be more disciplined with your thoughts, words, and actions. Saint Paul tells the Hebrews that as a Christian, "there will be trials you will need to suffer for the sake of being a disciple" (Heb 12:7).

So instead of giving up when things get hard or letting your mind play tricks on you, such as telling yourself that you 'can't', you need to flip the script. Instead of giving up, try again and use positive words that encourage and motivate you to keep moving towards the goal. If the goal is to become a better disciple, then you are going to need to be more disciplined. It is not easy to be a disciple, you need to be countercultural. This word, countercultural is used often in the writings of Matthew Kelly creator of the *Dynamic Catholic Institute*. It is a reminder that God's ways are not the ways of the world and as a disciple you will need to shift your thinking to see things through God's eyes.

The experiences of *Discipleship 5K*, give you the opportunity to do the work of becoming a better disciple. It requires discipline both physically and spiritually to become stronger and build endurance. Think about the words, *disciple* and *discipline*. There are only two extra letters in discipline, *I* and *N*. When you use discipline, consider yourself IN training to become a disciple; perhaps this shift in thinking will help you see the time and effort you put into *Discipleship 5K* a little differently.

JOURNAL

Your mind can play tricks on you, but you can override these thoughts of not feeling worthy or good enough. It takes practice but you can do it. Just remember to see yourself through God's eyes and He made you worthy and good.

Name a few things that might be tricking you into thinking this challenge was not such a clever idea?

Name a few ways you feel defeated in your daily life?

Write down the negative words you tell yourself.

Encourage three people today. When you encourage others, you give them words to battle those negative thoughts in their heads. Encouraging others is a fantastic way to help you feel encouraged too. It is good to practice what you want to say by writing it down so your thoughts and intention can be clear. Writing it down is only part of the process, be sure to follow through by encouraging those whom you chose to encourage. Your words may be the only positive words they hear today and can make a big difference. Write down who you want to encourage and what you will say to them.

Today I will encourage…
by saying…

Today I will encourage…
by saying…

Today I will encourage…
by saying…

ACTION

As you move your body, use the words of encouragement you wrote for others as your mantra this week to keep you motivated and to push yourself a little harder. Tell yourself you are strong. Tell yourself you are worthy. Tell yourself you can achieve your goals.

Before you walk or run, spend 5-10 minutes stretching and do another 5-10 minutes of calisthenics to warm up before your walk or run.

Level 1: walk ½- ¾ a mile as fast as you can
Level 2: run 1-2.5 miles at your peak pace
Level 3: run 2.5-6 miles at your peak pace

Stronger Together

Scripture: Esther 3:1-7

> Set his seat above all the officials who were with him. (Esth 3:1).

REFLECTION

Mordecai did not want to bow down to the new king because he was a Jew and knew it was against God's Law to put someone above God. This was unacceptable to the king so, Haman, the king, vowed to kill all the Jews in the kingdom.

People today still act this way. It seems everyone wants to make themselves out to be more powerful than another person, and if the people do not comply, then they turn violent. Scenarios like this have played out many times throughout history because of different religious beliefs, like in the Scripture or because someone is of a different race, gender, or economic status.

Do not allow others to narrate your story. When someone wants you to do something you know is wrong, makes you feel like you do not belong, do not accept you for who you are or because of what you believe, do not let their hurtful words or actions keep you from doing what you know is right. When you face these challenges, remember you are part of something bigger than yourself because you are a child of God, and He has a plan for you.

It takes a lot of courage to stand up alone, but Mordecai was not alone. He had all his fellow Jews who also believed what he believed. You are not alone either. You are a part of a team of disciples who are called to make a difference in the world. Although there may be times when you must stand up alone, you can have confidence that when you are standing up for what is right and what is just, others will follow. Those who have common goals and values work together to make a greater impact; there are examples that throughout history too.

JOURNAL

The same goes for this *Discipleship 5K* journey. You are not alone in this challenge; you are a part of the team of disciples who are working to be stronger both physically and spiritually. So, even if you began this journey on your own, you can know that there are others who are working towards the same goal. Additionally, there are people who are being a witness to your strength and determination to do something good for yourself by taking part in the challenge. Some of these people may even be inspired by the commitment you made and are making different choices in their own physical and spiritual development. Go out and make a difference!

> Identify some of those people who are standing with you, who have noticed how you are making a difference in your life physically and spiritually.

It is one thing to make positive changes within yourself to show you are a disciple, but it is another thing to step out in your discipleship to do something for others. Think of areas in your life where you need to come together with someone who is already making a difference and consider a little way you can help make a significant difference. Perhaps you are already a part of a team of people working together to do something positive.

Write down what team or teams you are currently a member, for example, a task force at work, as member of a church community, a book club, or a fan of a sports team.

How do you express your membership?

How does it make you feel to be a member of this group?

How does your membership have a positive impact on your life and/or in the community?

ACTION

Try to breathe in for 5 seconds, hold the breath for 5 seconds and release the breath for 5 seconds.

Level 1: take a break from physical activity but spend time breathing with your eyes closed as you reflect on the journal questions
Level 2: spend 15-20 minutes doing yoga or stretching
Level 3: spend 30-60 minutes of yoga or stretching

God's Image

Scripture: Genesis 1:26-31

> God created mankind in his image, in the image of
> God he created them; male and female he created
> them. (Gen 1:27)

REFLECTION

The scripture passage from the first chapter of Genesis is a message of how God created all things, but He paid special attention to creating humankind. "God looked at all He created and said it was good, then looked at humanity, which was created in His image, and said it was very good" (Gen 1:26-31, author's paraphrase). Your challenge today is to see yourself as God sees you, as very good.

Sometimes you might think you are not good enough to do something. Maybe you are not able to keep up with the physical or spiritual training of *Discipleship 5K* and you think you might as well just give up. Perhaps you let negative thoughts creep into your head that trick you into thinking you are not good enough; or that you look stupid or funny when you run and are embarrassed because you sweat. These thoughts are not from God. God created you in His own image, everyone; old or young, chubby or skinny, tall or short, and He loves every little dimple on your thigh and freckle on your nose.

God knows you better than you know yourself. He sees you as very good. You may not always feel that way and there might be parts of you that you do not like, but God loves you just the same. There are people in your life who love you just the way you are too!

JOURNAL

Write a love letter to yourself, from God.

ACTION

Take time today to do your breathing exercises. Think about how your breath comes from God and allow your thoughts to be consumed by God. The love God has for you is unconditional and everlasting. You are loved!

Level 1: walk 1-2 miles at a moderate pace
Level 2: jog 2-4 miles at a moderate pace
Level 3: run 3-7 miles at a moderate pace

DAY 11

Mental Toughness

Scripture: Joshua 24:1-28

> As for me and my household, we will serve the Lord.
> (Josh 24:15)

REFLECTION

Joshua has a tough task ahead of him and this piece of scripture reflects what you have ahead of you. It takes discipline to be a disciple, and this means building up mental toughness to be able to endure conflicts that arise. Joshua 24:15 says, "as for me and my household, we will serve the Lord," which is a reminder to choose God, even if there are people tempting you to deviate from your plan. You need to build up the mental toughness to stand up for what you believe and continue to work towards your goals.

At almost two weeks into the challenge, this passage could be just what you need to hear. You might be facing some of your own temptations to turn away from doing the work of *Discipleship 5K* which you have committed to do and fall back into your old ways. It can be difficult on you to do the physical and/or spiritual activities but it may also be having an impact on some of your relationships. Maybe even in a negative way. There could be some family or friends who are upset because your participation in this challenge has affected the time you spend with them or maybe the way you spend time with them has changed.

When you encounter struggles in relationships you should not just give up. There will be differences of priorities and opinions in all relationships and learning how to navigate through the difficult times is one of life's biggest challenges. If everyone agreed on everything all the time, then life would be a little boring. The value of relationships is simply too great to break ties with everyone you ever disagree with or because you have different interests. Shutting people out or down because of conflicts or differences in priorities could cause you to end up all alone and that is not good for your physical, spiritual, or even emotional heath. It is important to have an honest conversation about what you are doing and why you are doing it so the people in your life understand that some of these changes might be permanent.

It is possible that you have not encountered any conflicts with others as you go through the exercises of *Discipleship 5K*, instead your conflict is within yourself. You can be your own biggest obstacle by allowing negative thoughts and other people's opinions to make decisions for your life. It is necessary to put into practice some ways to keep the negativity from gaining momentum and keeping you from achieving your goals. Turn to God to help you squash those negative thoughts inside your head before they grow into a problem.

Think of a toddler who is just beginning to learn to walk. They fall so many times and incur bumps and bruises along the way. You never hear of a toddler who gives up and decides they will simply crawl for the rest of their lives because they do not learn to walk right away. Instead, they continue to persevere because they do not know quitting is an option.

So, when you are out there doing your physical training and your body tells you that you just cannot go anymore, reach out to God to come help you overcome your weakness. Allow God to give you the strength you need to train your mind and heart to make it that extra mile. Trust that God will pull you through and you do not have the option to quit. Your heart already knows how to trust God, it is time to train your mind to do the same.

JOURNAL

You need a game plan. This is what professional athletes do to prepare for competition, they imagine the worst-case scenario situations and find the best course of action. Today, you will do the same.

> Write down specific tasks or actions you will put into practice when your mind and or body tells you that you are ready to quit a physical exercise.

> Write down specific things you will do to help keep the spiritual goals you have set forth. You are battling old habits and creating new ones, create a plan to help yourself be successful.

ACTION

The next time you feel you cannot go any further, push yourself to not stop until you reach the next mailbox or the next driveway or the next quarter/half mile. Mental toughness is required for both running and discipleship.

Level 1: do 15-20 minutes of a cross-training activity
Level 2: do 30-45 minutes of a cross-training activity
Level 3: do 60-90 minutes of a cross-training activity

Perseverance Pays

Scripture: Ruth 4:14-17

He shall be to you a restorer of life. (Ruth 4:15)

REFLECTION

This scripture tells the end of the story of Boaz and Ruth. What you need to know is that Ruth journeyed into a foreign land as a peasant woman and Boaz was a wealthy person. Boaz and Ruth got married despite their many differences in the eyes of the community. Their union was an outward sign of how God's love shows no partiality and sees through race and economic differences. Boaz and Ruth showed much faithfulness and integrity when following God's Will and they were blessed with a son who became the father of Jesse, the father of David. If you know much about salvation history, David is the bloodline of Jesus.

Sometimes you might get discouraged and feel like the world is against you, someone does not like you, or you are discriminated against for some reason or another. This is no reason to give up. God has a plan for you, a great plan. You need to stick to your path and continue to fight on in faithfulness. Ruth from the Bible is a perfect example of someone who stuck with something even though it was hard. God rewarded her because she persevered through some tough times and God will reward you too.

JOURNAL

Ruth is someone who did the right thing over and over, then God rewarded her for doing what was right. Maybe you need a little of Ruth's perseverance right about now. It is time to check in with yourself. Do not get discouraged. God has a plan for you. He will take care of you as long as you remain faithful to your task.

> Describe how you feel when you lay down at the end of the night to go to bed after you have completed your physical and spiritual exercises with *Discipleship 5K*.

> Describe how you feel on the nights you do not do your physical or spiritual training.

> Write a review of how your training is going so far both physically and spiritually. Are you on the right path and staying faithful to the original goal?

Write down how you feel about your efforts both physically and spiritually. Are you doing all you can or is there room for improvement?

ACTION

Perseverance pays! Stick with it! Add in a little extra today by doing 10 minutes of calisthenics in addition to your scheduled exercise.

Level 1: do 10-15 minutes of yoga or stretching
Level 2: do 10-15 minutes of yoga or stretching and run 1-2.5 miles at your peak pace
Level 3: do 10-15 minutes of yoga or stretching and run 2.5-6 miles at your peak pace

DAY 13

Open to Change

Scripture: 1 Corinthians 1:10-17

> Be united in the same mind and the purpose.
> (1 Cor 1:10)

REFLECTION

As you prepare for this race, it is really preparing you to be a changed person inside and out. It is not easy to change but it becomes easier when you know you do not have to go through it alone. The obstacles may be new to you, but the scripture passages you read throughout the challenge identify people in the Bible who have faced these obstacles too. You can see how they were able to overcome these obstacles with God's help and learn from them.

Take the scripture from Saint Paul to the Corinthians you read today, the early Christians got distracted from the common goal and began to get petty by trying to do what was best for themselves and not for the greater good. This could be you, getting distracted from the goal of being dedicated to working on your physical and spiritual health and deciding you would rather snuggle up in your recliner and fall into a Netflix coma.

Remember earlier this week when you read the scripture about Joshua who was trying to get everyone to arrive at the goal the same way but realized the most important thing was that they served God. Maybe you are having a tough time staying motivated with the physical activities and are afraid to go off course. Learn from Joshua and do not get tripped up by the details. Change it up, it is your challenge and only you know you best. Maybe you need to walk at a new park, or you need to swap a rest day for a workout day because you have a date night, parent teacher conference, or a work event and your schedule will not allow an hour walk. Joshua learned he needed to be flexible and allow himself some grace. This is a good lesson to learn through this process, to be kind to yourself and accept some of God's grace when things do not work out the way you had planned.

Then there is the spiritual side. You might find it hard to carve out time in your day to dive into the scripture and reflect. This is not a new conflict. Anyone who has made the commitment to dive into a deeper relationship with Jesus, has come up against opposition. Just like with the exercises, you need to switch it up. Sometimes what you think will work one day will not work the next. Your prayer time is supposed to come away feeling rested and peaceful, not anxious and frustrated.

It is okay to do things differently, you do not have to do the same thing all the time. The only consistency you need, is to show up and give your best every day. This is when you can be like Ruth and continue to move forward, trying to do the right thing, again and again. Do not let a minor excuse get in the way of your physical or spiritual training, make the necessary changes so you will be successful.

JOURNAL

Make a list of things that distract you from your focus of training for the 5K and your discipleship training.

Name things that could distract you from your physical goal.

Name things that could distract you from your spiritual goal.

Brainstorm ideas to help motivate you to remain focused. What might you need to change to stay on the right path?

ACTION

Stay the course. Be persistent. Nothing worth doing is easy. Be sure to schedule time to stretch before and after your walk or jog.

Level 1: take a 1–2-mile leisurely walk
Level 2: take a 3–5-mile leisurely walk
Level 3: take a 3–5-mile leisurely jog

Believe

Scripture: Mark 9:14-29

> This kind can come out only through prayer (Mark 9:29).

REFLECTION

The Gospel story about Jesus casting out demons of a young boy is important. The family wants Jesus to heal the boy because they heard that He could. Jesus does not want the family to just ask Jesus because they are desperate to save their son, He wants them to believe in Him.

Saying you believe in something may not be enough to prove you genuinely believe. You might still have a twinge of doubt about whether you can really go through with this challenge. You might not believe that God can really help you through the physical part of the training. One of the toughest tests of faith is letting go of control and trusting God to come through. When God answers prayers, the outcome may not be what you wanted, but it always goes according to God's plan.

Imagine Jesus is here right now. Is there something you want Him to exorcise from you? Open yourself up in prayer and ask God to remove any stress or pain you feel. When you tell God through prayer how you feel and ask Him to help you in the struggle, He will do it. You must let it go first.

Today, put your faith into action and during your stretching and yoga, focus on connecting to God through your breathing. While you are breathing and moving, ask God to remove any obstacles that are slowing you down or keeping you from doing your best in the challenge. God will take it from here, you just need to hand it over to Him.

JOURNAL

What you say is not nearly as important as *how* you say it. Your attitude makes a difference. Jesus wants to know that you believe He will help you when you are down, not just because you say so, but because it is spoken through your actions too.

> Write down how God is showing up for you in your physical challenge.

> Write down how God is showing up for you in your spiritual challenge.

> Write down the ways you reflect God in the challenge.

ACTION

Try to be mindful of how it feels when your body is full of air and how it feels differently when it is empty. Reflect how it is similar to how you feel when you feel God's presence near you and when you do not feel close to God.

Level 1: take a day to rest and spend 5 minutes working on your breathing
Level 2: do 15-20 minutes of yoga or stretching and 20-40 minutes of a cross-training activity
Level 3: do 20-40 minutes of yoga or stretching and 30-60 minutes of a cross-training activity

WEEK TWO OVERVIEW

Write down any thoughts, words of encouragement, ideas for growth or measurements of progress you have from this week from your physical and spiritual training.

WEEK THREE
Tools for the Spiritual Journey

You need to gather up your tools for the spiritual journey. Start the week off with inspiration from your favorite authors, prayer books and scripture. It can be in the form of an inspirational quote, a family motto, or a Bible verse but this week you will add tools you need to stay motivated on the journey. These words can help you grow spiritually but also motivate you when you are feeling tired or weak. This week you will focus on prayer and practice leaning on God to help you though, even when you think it is impossible.

Stay the Course

Scripture: 2 Chronicles 32:27-33

> God left him to himself, in order to test him and to
> know all that was in his heart. (2 Chr 32:31)

REFLECTION

Today is the start of week three and it is time to step up your efforts
a little more. Each week of *Discipleship 5K* is meant to challenge you
to see how much more you can do. If you simply go through the
motions of the physical and spiritual activities, you might reach the
goal of completing the challenge, but you will not be changed. To
become a better disciple, you need to put your heart and soul into
the activities too, so you can build the strength you need to persevere
when the road gets rough.

In society today, people start projects and get distracted and lose
interest. This happens when obtaining a college degree, finding a
job and even in long-term personal relationships. When there is a
conflict or you no longer have interest, it is easier to run away than
to face the situation and try to fix the problem. This mindset will
not help you on this challenge.

One of the goals of the *Discipleship 5K* is to help you change
your mindset so when things get tough and you think you should
quit, you will persevere instead. Perseverance is a valuable skill which
everyone can benefit from and is the key ingredient to many of the
mega hit movies such as, the Star Wars Saga and Marvel's Avenger
Series. The characters refuse to stop moving towards their goal when
faced with obstacles and challenges.

Yes, you will get discouraged and lose heart when you are asked to do hard things during this challenge, but it is training for life. When you practice perseverance, you will be ready when demanding situations come your way. Look to Hezekiah for assurance that God will reward you for the good you do. Stay on course, press on, and you will see the benefits begin to unfold.

JOURNAL

Remember a time when you wanted to quit but a friend or family member told you to persevere and keep going. Write them a thank you note and let them know you still appreciate their support. Perhaps they need a few words of encouragement today and your note will put a smile on their face.

> Write your note here to practice what you want to say. Then when you look back you can be encouraged by your words of gratitude.

ACTION

As you stretch, think about what you will write in the thank you note. Do 10-20 minutes of calisthenics before or after your walk or run.

> Level 1: walk ¾-1 mile as fast as you can
> Level 2: run 1-2.5 miles at your peak pace
> Level 3: run 2.5-6 miles at your peak pace

Come Holy Spirit

Scripture: Hebrews 10:36

> For you need endurance, so that when you have
> done the will of God, you may receive what was
> promised.

REFLECTION

Scripture says you need endurance to do the Will of God. Through the challenge, you are taking care of yourself physically which might mean it is helping you sleep better or to choose healthier snacks. You are also spending designated time in prayer, talking to God with intention, which might inspire you to be more loving, compassionate, or patient with yourself and others.

You need endurance to be a disciple but sometimes there are things that slow you down. You might get frustrated and impatient or overreact to situations and let your impulsiveness get you into trouble. There could be times when you act out by being sarcastic or feel someone is attacking you, so you get defensive. When you feel your patience going and you feel as if you cannot go one more step, you need to call on the Holy Spirit. When you do, you will be filled with what you need to continue, to persevere. Take time to literally breathe in the Holy Spirit before the humanness takes over, you do not have to do it alone.

JOURNAL

The Holy Spirit gives the best gifts. They are wisdom, counsel, fortitude, knowledge, understanding, piety, and fear of the Lord. You will need each of these at some point in your life or through this challenge. Today reflect on each of them and choose just one to ask the Holy Spirit to bring it to you to help in a specific situation. Perhaps you need one of the gifts to help you on this journey of *Discipleship 5K* or maybe you need one of the gifts to help you with a personal relationship or a work project. Whatever gift you need, and for whatever reason, accept the gift.

> Write a prayer to the Holy Spirit to say thank you and hand over the stress and anxiety you carry because of that issue. Ask the Holy Spirit for the gift(s) you need to help you stay on track with your goals.

ACTION

Choose one of the gifts of the Holy Spirit to focus on and help you through the exercise today.

> Level 1: spend 15-20 minutes doing a cross-training activity
> Level 2: pend 30-45 minutes doing a cross-training activity
> Level 3: spend 60-90 minutes doing a cross-training activity

DAY 17

It is Not All About You

Scripture: Galatians 6:2

> Bear one another's burdens, and in this way you will fulfill the law of Christ.

REFLECTION

Sometimes when you are dealing with something you think you are all alone in the struggle. You forget Jesus sent the disciples out two by two so they might have a companion on the journey. You too have companions on the journey.

Make a point to find someone who is in a similar place as you; either in trying a new routine or training for a 5K. It could be a person from work, someone who you sit by on the bus, or perhaps the person who greets you as you come to church. Whether you are making great strides in your 5K training or if you are struggling, you need to reach out to others who are on the same path as you. Part of being a disciple is getting comfortable enough to reach out to others and invite them on the journey. They could need to be encouraged and you can help build them up.

Saint Paul tells the Galatians to bear one another's burdens. It is a reminder that you are not alone in the world and that God calls everyone to be Christ to one another. The world preaches a different message, but you are not of this world, you are a disciple. You know God's ways are not the ways of the world, so when the world says it is all about you, it is wrong. A big part of being a disciple is walking the walk with others. This means you need to reach out to others and share the faith, this is evangelization.

JOURNAL

When you reach out to others for no other reason than to check in with them, it can lift their spirits and it is a good reminder that the world is not all about you.

> Make a list of people you need to reach out to and share a word of encouragement or just let them know you are there for them if they need anything.

ACTION

Be sure to focus on the stretch and your body/soul connection to God through the stretch. Spend time stretching before and after your walk, jog, or run.

> Level 1: walk 1-2 miles at a moderate pace
> Level 2: jog 2-4 miles at a moderate pace
> Level 3: run 3-7 miles at a moderate pace

God is Here

Scripture: Psalm 77:1

> I cry aloud to God, aloud to God, that he may hear me.

REFLECTION

When you began this training, you might have thought it was a great idea. Now after a few weeks you might be rethinking the commitment you made. You need to remember you are not alone in this. Not only do you need to seek the company and support of others who are on this path, but you also need to reach out to God. You need to call out to God in prayer.

The scripture from Psalms today says to cry out to God. This means sometimes you need to speak to God out loud and not just in your head. Speak to God as though He is right in front of you having a conversation. People complain that God is not there or He is not listening, but the communication barrier is not coming from God. Instead, the barrier comes from the thought that God already knows everything, so what is the point of telling Him. However, God wants you to share your life with Him and that includes sharing your joys and struggles in your prayer.

When you pray, you acknowledge God's presence in your life. You are a child of God and a member of the faith community, and you are loved. God communicates this through prayer, in response to what you share with Him. When you share your joys and struggles with God in prayer, it can give you clarity of mind and it allows you the time and space to be open for a response. God is waiting to hear what you need so He can shower you with love, grace, and mercy.

JOURNAL

God is in the good and in the bad. Talk to God, being honest about how you feel and what you need. End each prayer by expressing your love and gratitude for all He does for you.

Write a prayer to God telling Him of your struggles.

Write a prayer to God telling Him of your joys.

ACTION

Imagine as you breathe today, inhaling God's goodness and exhaling stress and negativity.

Level 1: take a day to rest and spend 5 minutes practicing breathing and connecting with God through your breathing exercises

Level 2: do 15-20 minutes of yoga or stretching and 20-40 minutes of a cross-training activity

Level 3: do 20-40 minutes of yoga or stretching and 30-60 minutes of a cross-training activity

DAY 19

Three Words

Scripture: Psalm 18:2

> The Lord is my rock, my fortress, and my deliverer,
> my God, my rock in whom I take refuge, my shield,
> and the horn of my salvation, my stronghold.

REFLECTION

The scripture passage from the book of Psalms describes God as a rock, a fortress, and a deliverer. These are powerful words. They describe God as a strong protector who provides shelter from whatever might come. This is how the author of the book of Psalms described God.

Since God is all things to all people, He can be described in a million other ways too. Even in your lifetime, you might describe God differently at different times, depending on what you are experiencing in your life. Today, take time to brainstorm the words you use to describe God right now.

As you continue to do the work physically and spiritually on this challenge, remember the words of the scripture, especially on those days that cause you a little trouble. God is there to help you if you need it, and He is ready, willing, and able to deliver you to your goal.

JOURNAL

Words can hold a lot of meaning and today the words from the scripture describe an amazing image of God. These words hold specific meaning to the person who wrote Psalm 18; it is how they describe who God is for them. Today, you will determine what words you will use to describe God. Choose three words to describe God and then name three words you would use to identify yourself. When you pick words, remember to use adjectives that describe you and not use the nouns that describe your roles, i.e., wife, mother, etc. If you find it difficult to describe yourself, consider what words God would use to describe you.

Three words to describe God.

Three words to describe yourself.

ACTION

While doing the exercise today, put forth the effort you believe God wants you to put forth.

Level 1: spend at least 15 minutes taking part in a cross-training activity

Level 2: spend at least 30 minutes taking part in a cross-training activity

Level 3: spend at least 45 minutes taking part in a cross-training activity

DAY 20

Thank God

Scripture: Philippians 1:3

I thank my God every time I remember you.

REFLECTION

In the Catholic tradition at the end of Mass, the congregation says, "Thanks be to God." This is communicated at the end to express gratitude to God. When you pray, much of what you do is to thank God for life and for those you love. It is a good practice to give thanks to God but also to show gratitude to those around you.

The scripture for today says, "I thank my God every time I remember you" (Phil 1:3). You could make a lengthy list of people for whom you are grateful to God for having in your life, especially those who encourage and inspire you to be a better person. Some may have literally given birth to you, some you have known your whole life, some you never met, and some may no longer be living here on earth. There is not a statute of limitations on the people you can be grateful to for making an impact on your life.

It is time you express gratitude for those people and reflect on the attributes they have for which you are grateful. Of course, you are grateful for God and your family, but today the challenge is to look beyond your normal 'go to' people. Do not limit yourself to only people who are living or that you have met in person but consider those whose words or actions inspired you in a unique way.

JOURNAL

Thank God for the people in your life whom you admire and who inspire you. You draw strength from God and from others to be the person you were created to be. As you write the names of the people you are grateful for, also list the traits you admire about them. Remember, they can be alive or dead, so long as they have been a role model to you and affected your life.

> I am grateful for…
> because…

> I am grateful for…
> because…

> I am grateful for…
> because…

If you do not already know who your patron saint is, take time to look it up. A patron saint is someone who has the same name as you such as Christopher or Katherine. If you do not have a patron saint, you can find out who the saint of the day is today and read their biography. Further, you can search for the patron saint of different occupations or interests such as doctors or cooking. Search for the patron saint of runners and pray to them to help you while you train. Write down what you learn.

My Patron Saint is…

How am I inspired by him/her and how can his/
her life experience change my life in a positive way?

ACTION

Make sure to do some light stretching before and after your walk or
jog. Remember to breathe deeply as you stretch.

> Level 1: take a 1–2-mile leisurely walk
> Level 2: take a 3–5-mile leisurely walk
> Level 3: take a 3–5-mile leisurely jog

DAY 21

Power of Prayer

Scripture: Matthew 6:7

When you are praying, do not heap up empty phrases as the Gentiles do; for they think that they will be heard because of their many words.

REFLECTION

When you pray, many times you pray the memorized prayers you have known since childhood and there is nothing wrong with these prayers. However, as you grow in your discipleship, you should begin to use your own words to express your thoughts and your needs. There are people in your families and community who need prayer, and you can pray for them by either praying one of the memorized prayers on their behalf or by using your own words. Prayer is powerful; you should make sure you are giving it the respect and attention it deserves.

If you believe words are powerful, then it is only natural to believe prayer is powerful too since prayer is a series of words. When you pray, it is important to be mindful of your words and not just say things to be heard or to sound important. Be specific with your words in your prayers and let what you believe lead your words because your words lead your actions.

JOURNAL

Let your words have meaning, pray with feeling and be specific. Make a goal to pray for least five people or situations. If you are not sure who to pray for, watch the news or ask to be added to a prayer chain list at church. You have the power to pray powerful prayers. God's waiting to hear from you.

Name of the person or situation you will pray for today.

Write your specific prayer.

Name of the person or situation you will pray for today.

Write your specific prayer.

Name of the person or situation you will pray for today.

Write your specific prayer.

Name of the person or situation you will pray for today.

Write your specific prayer.

Name of the person or situation you will pray for today.

Write your specific prayer.

ACTION

Say a prayer with each cycle of your inhale and exhale. Remember the physical activity suggested is only a suggestion and if you want to take a rest, then do it. Listen to what your body needs to remain in the race.

Level 1: rest from physical activity but practice breathing for 10 minutes
Level 2: spend 15-20 minutes practicing your breathing and do 20-40 minutes of a cross-training activity

Level 3: spend 15-20 minutes practicing your breathing and do 30-60 minutes of a cross-training activity

WEEK THREE OVERVIEW

Write down any thoughts, words of encouragement, ideas for growth or measurements of progress you have from this week from your physical and spiritual training.

WEEK FOUR
Change Will Do You Good

Congratulations, you are still here! Whether you have found a groove or gotten into a rut, it is time to introduce new exercises or hit a new trail. This week is about staying motivated as you come to the end of the first month of the challenge. You do not want to get bored with your exercise routine because if you are uninterested in doing the workout, the likelihood of reaching the goal is null. Find a new park to take your walk, ask a friend or co-worker if they will join you for a yoga or kick-boxing class at the community center, or download a new exercise app on your phone or tablet; the goal is to mix it up so you can look forward to your exercise time.

Prophetic Frenzy

Scripture: 1 Samuel 10:6

> Then the Spirit of the Lord will possess you, and
> you will be in a prophetic frenzy along with them
> and be turned into a different person.

REFLECTION

'Prophetic Frenzy' are the words used in the scripture today to describe a person filled with the Holy Spirit. This describes you. You are a different person because you are aware that you are filled with the Holy Spirit and the fruits of your labor are shining through.

The work you have done both physically and spiritually are beginning to show. You are becoming a new creation, not only on the outside but you are also different on the inside. There is evidence of your discipline and hard work. Perhaps you are feeling more energetic, or your muscles are not as sore as before which allows you to go faster or further in your workouts. This piece of scripture is a great motivator to continue the good work that has begun within you.

JOURNAL

Create goals for the next few weeks to help stay motivated. Here are a couple of suggestions:

1. Think back to people who have encouraged you and remember their words.

2. Ask someone to pray for you as you hit this milestone of one month of your *Discipleship 5K* journey.

Reflect on how you have changed since you began the training.

Write your goals.

ACTION

Even though your goal is to walk or run in a 5K, you need to work on building other muscle groups too. Spend 5-10 minutes before or after your walk or run doing calisthenics.

Level 1: walk ¾-1 mile as fast as you can
Level 2: run 1-2.5 miles at your peak pace
Level 3: run 2.5-6 miles at your peak pace

DAY 23

Partners of Christ

Scripture: Hebrews 3:13

> But exhort one another everyday, as long as it is
> called "today," so that none of you may be hardened
> by the deceitfulness of sin. (Heb 3:13)

REFLECTION

Saint Paul is calling you to lift up your neighbor and be Christ for
them. And he says, do it today, do not wait until tomorrow. "Take
care, Brothers and Sisters...for we have become partners of Christ."
(Heb 3:12,14), these words are sandwiched between the scripture for
today. When you read Hebrews 3:12-14, it clearly says it is the job
of all disciples to help one another.

You are called to help build the Kingdom of God and one of
the best ways to do this is to encourage one another, to build each
other up. Jesus is the perfect role model. He went from city to city
spending time with the people. He often healed someone of what
was troubling them, simply by touching them. You have this power
too. Sometimes when you spend time with another person, hold
their hand or give them a hug, it can bring them peace and comfort
them. That is powerful! Today you may be the only example of
Jesus another person sees, so you must go out there and let your
light shine brightly.

JOURNAL

Invite a friend to join you for your physical activity today. It is a wonderful way to have fun and spend time together. If that is not possible or if you want to do a bonus activity, walk or run to a friend's house for a visit. It might be someone who cannot get out and needs to be reminded that they are loved, or it could be someone you have not seen for a while, and you just want to stop to say hello.

Also, remember to keep praying for those people who need prayer, especially anyone new you heard about in the news who is struggling. You do not have to know the person to pray for them; remember they are your brother or sister in Christ.

> Write down what you decide to do and then write down how the experience felt for both you and your partner in Christ.

ACTION

Step out of your comfort zone and try something new. Remember to stretch before you begin your activity.

> Level 1: spend at least 15 minutes taking part in a new cross-training activity
> Level 2: spend at least 30 minutes taking part in a new cross-training activity
> Level 3: spend at least 45 minutes taking part in a new cross-training activity

DAY 24
Simply Be

Scripture: Psalm 139:23

> Search me, O God, and know my heart; test me and
> know my thoughts.

REFLECTION

God knows when you sit and when you stand. He knows when you
are obedient to His word and when you fill your days with other
things. Thank goodness God is not keeping a tally sheet of the times
you choose to spend doing other things rather than doing what He
calls you to do.

It is important to schedule time to simply *be* with God. It helps
bring your body, mind, and spirit together when you slow down and
breathe. Set aside time to be silent today and allow God to be with
you and just you. Give God your full attention. Breathe. Be still.
Connect with God. This is the goal for today.

JOURNAL

Today, spend time alone with God. Make a point to sit down and
spend time in silence. Do not say or think, simply be. Push all the
distractions out of your mind and try to relax. When you have done
this, write down some notes from the experience.

What is easy or difficult to be silent and simply be?

What suggestions do you have for the next time? Will there be a next time?

Write whatever comes to mind so you can remember the experience.

ACTION

Do not turn on meditative music today, just sit in silence. Allow God to speak to you. Close your eyes and make space within your body for Him through your breathing. Imagine breathing God in with each inhalation and blowing out negativity, stress, worry, and any thoughts that are not of God or of the present moment. Practice making room for God in the activity for today.

> Level 1: take a day of rest from physical activity but push yourself to spend up to 10 minutes in silence and focus on breathing in God's presence
> Level 2: practice 15-20 minutes of yoga or stretching and do 20-40 minutes of a cross-training activity
> Level 3: practice 20-40 minutes of yoga or stretching and do 30-60 minutes of a cross-training activity

No Pity Parties

Scripture: James 1:2-4

> Because you know that the testing of your faith
> produces endurance. (Jas 1:3)

REFLECTION

Every day brings its own set of obstacles, expectations, and obligations. There might be days when you feel you cannot keep up. There could be days when you struggle with meeting the expectations of others or of yourself. Just because you fall a few steps behind does not mean you need to quit the race. You are still alive and have a goal to get to the cross.

Take a deep breath. Do the best you can by being okay with your progress, even if it is not where you think you are supposed to be. You need to accept that there will be times when you are distracted by life and do not show up the way you want to. These are times when your strength and dedication are tested. Do not let a few steps back make you give up. God gives you a clean slate every day to begin again and you can begin fresh every day with the activities of *Discipleship 5K* too.

God knows you and knows you are enough, you are worthy, and you are capable. He knows because He made you that way. The voice in your head can sometimes drown out God's voice, so today in your prayer time you will do an activity to alleviate the negatives and turn them into positives. You can do it. Believe in yourself the way God believes in you.

JOURNAL

Doubt. Hesitation. Suspicion. Distrust. These things are not of God and when you let them in, you can get detoured from your goals. Negativity can choke out the good fruit you have produced if you let it.

Write down each negative thought that tempts you to throw yourself a pity party on its own piece of paper, an index card or a post-it note. Once you have written down all your negative thoughts, throw the paper on the ground and stomp on it, then pick it up and rip it into itty bitty pieces. Each time you tear the paper, say a positive word or phrase as though God is speaking directly to you. What words would God say to you, or about you, that would battle the negative thoughts you have been thinking? When you are finished throw the pieces away OR put them in a container; somewhere you will be able to see them each day. Do not let these feelings of doubt creep in and spoil the victory you have ahead of you.

> Write the negative thoughts and positive words here so you can look back on them when you need encouragement.

> Negative   Positive

Write down your thoughts and feelings about this activity so you can look back on the experience.

ACTION

In addition to your walk or run, do 10 minutes of calisthenics before or after your run.

Level 1: walk ¾-1 mile as fast as you can
Level 2: run 1-2.5 miles at your peak pace
Level 3: run 2.5-6 miles at your peak pace

DAY 26

Greater Purpose

Scripture: Romans 8:28

> We know that all things work together for good for
> those who love God, who are called according to
> his purpose.

REFLECTION

There are times when you feel like the road ahead is an uphill
climb and you can get discouraged. In these moments you need
to remember you are called to a greater purpose as a follower and
disciple of Christ. You are not the first, nor will you be the last
person to face these uphill climbs. There is a point in everyone's life,
even Jesus,' when you get to a point where the path before you seems
overwhelming. God does not leave you alone to face these struggles,
He is there with you every step of the way.

God is there ready, willing, and able to walk every step of the
journey with you. Seek God and open yourself up to the work He
is doing in your life. When you made the decision to begin this
journey, you had a clear focus. Go back and revisit that focus to see
how you are doing. If you need to adjust your focus, that is okay.
You need a clear focus if you want to increase the likelihood of
completing your goal. It is time to get re-connected to your purpose.

JOURNAL

Remember what motivated you to start the *Discipleship 5K* in the first place? Are those things still what motivate you?

Do you feel stronger physically and spiritually? Explain.

Write down three ways God is specifically showing up to help you be successful on your path to discipleship.

Then give thanks to God for being there to support you and motivate you, and yes, sometimes carry you. Express your gratitude in prayer, telling God thank you for being there for you when you need. Write your prayer here.

ACTION

God is in your breath because He is the one who breathed life into you. Remember to breathe deeply as you do your exercise and reflect on ways God is showing up for you.

> Level 1: do 10-15 minutes of yoga or stretching
> Level 2: do 20-30 minutes of a cross-training activity and spend 10-15 minutes doing a weight training activity
> Level 3: do 60-90 minutes of a cross-training activity and spend 15-20 minutes doing a weight training activity

DAY 27

Blessings

Scripture: Ephesians 1:3-4

> Blessed be the God and Father of our Lord Jesus Christ, who has blessed us in Christ with every spiritual blessing in the heavenly places. (Eph 1:3)

REFLECTION

Do not live life with blinders on your eyes. It is hard to recognize God everywhere and in everything, but He is there whether you see Him or not. Saint Paul is reminding the Ephesians that God has brought blessing to the world and the scripture is meant to remind you of this fact, too.

Find God in the trivial things and give thanks. It can sometimes be easier to see the things that go wrong, and they can distract you from seeing the blessings and gifts right in front of you. For example, the mere fact you woke up this morning is a gift from God. Whether the sun is shining, or it is raining; these are blessings, not just for you but for animals and for the earth. The food you eat, the clean water you drink or wash with are blessings that are too often taken for granted.

You have been given so much but it can easily be thought to be expected, instead of a blessing or a privilege. Do not let today pass by without recognizing God in the big things and the little things, then give Him praise. Thank you, God for all the blessings!

JOURNAL

Spend time thanking God for ALL of life's blessings as you do your physical training today and then complete the journal activity.

> Write down ten blessings, then twenty-five, and challenge yourself to find fifty ways God has blessed you just today.

ACTION

Take your time today during your exercise; you have a lot to think about. Do at least 10 minutes of stretching before and after your walk, do not rush through it.

> Level 1: take a 1.5-3-mile leisurely walk
> Level 2: take a 2–4-mile leisurely walk or jog
> Level 3: take a 4–6-mile leisurely walk or jog

DAY 28

Jesus is in the Boat

Scripture: Mark 4:41

> And they were filled with great awe and said to one another, "who then is this, that even the wind and the sea obey him."

REFLECTION

When you seek God, sometimes you can overlook Him, and think He is not there. But God is not playing hide and seek. He is in plain sight waiting for you to acknowledge Him. Do not fall into the trap of thinking God is not there or that you are not worthy to spend time with God because that is a lie from the devil. Remember yesterday's reflection reminded you that God is always present, even when you do not see Him.

The Disciples learned firsthand in the scripture from the Gospel of Mark, chapter 4, how important it is to turn to Jesus. They are in a boat in the middle of the sea when a storm rolls in, and the boat becomes unstable with the increasing winds and the high waves. In their fear and unrest, they wake Jesus up from His slumber. Jesus stands up, raises His hand, and says, "Peace! Be still!" (Mark 4:39) and the sea becomes calm again.

Jesus' presence and His words brought calm to the storm and removed the fear from the hearts of the Disciples. No matter what is going on in your life, Jesus is there. Sometimes you might wonder if He is present. You might get worried or scared and feel like you are alone, but like in this story from the scripture, when you call on Jesus, He can bring peace. Remember, Jesus is in the boat with you and ready, willing, and able to calm any storm that comes your way.

JOURNAL

Think of a time when you felt particularly close to God. Make a note of where you where, who was with you and how you felt. Sit in the presence of God for a few moments acknowledging His closeness to you. Today your goal is to connect deeply with that moment and try to carry the presence of God with you.

Write about your experience.

ACTION

Set the intention to seek God in every minute of your exercise and work to stay focused on God's presence as you do the activities.

Level 1: spend 15-20 minutes practicing yoga or stretching and 15-20 minutes doing a cross-training activity

Level 2: spend 20-30 minutes practicing yoga or stretching and 30-60 minutes doing a cross-training activity

Level 3: spend 30-60 minutes practicing yoga or stretching and 45-60 minutes doing a cross-training activity

WEEK FOUR OVERVIEW

Write down any thoughts, words of encouragement, ideas for growth or measurements of progress you have from this week from your physical and spiritual training.

WEEK FIVE
Celebrate Your Accomplishments

The definition of a disciple is someone who follows Jesus' teachings. Look back on how you have learned to be a better disciple over the past four weeks. There are so many things you have done to become a more devoted disciple by making your exercise time a priority and dedicating time with God in prayer; you should be so proud of yourself.

Celebrate your accomplishments thus far, but do not lose sight of what is still ahead of you. This past month you have been building the strength to persevere. Keep going! Do not get discouraged when you look forward, find ways to stay encouraged and keep the momentum going. Turn to God to help you push past the negative thoughts of 'I can't' and believe 'YOU CAN!' The scripture and journal exercise's this week will help you continue to make strides towards changing your mindset and build on the success you have already achieved.

DAY 29

God is Your Cheerleader

Scripture: Romans 8:31

> What then are we to say about these things? If God is for us, who is against us?

REFLECTION

There might be some doubt creeping into your mind as you begin the fifth week of this challenge, especially if you look ahead. Just because you are still two months away from the finish line, it is not an excuse to slow down. It may seem so far away, but you have made some great strides over the past four weeks, do not get discouraged or worry about the future.

The scripture today is encouraging you to press on because you have a secret weapon in your corner, God! Think about it, if God is for you, who can be against you? God is the Creator of the universe, Maker of all things and will not be defeated. These words of encouragement from Saint Paul were meant to motivate the Romans to stay focused on their task of spreading the Gospel to grow the kingdom of God. You can use these words from scripture today to remain focused on your goal, too.

It is encouraging to know you are not alone on this journey and that God is cheering you onto victory. You can be further encouraged, when you think that God is three in one, The Father, Son, and the Holy Spirit. The presence of the Holy Trinity really makes a powerful argument against slowing down now. You are just getting started and with the dream team behind you, there is no doubt you will complete the race.

JOURNAL

Imagine God the Father, Jesus, the Son, and the Holy Spirit in your corner or on the sidelines cheering you on and pushing you to do better and go further. Visualization is a great tool many high achievers use to do what some might deem impossible. When you visualize yourself doing it, you can go back anytime to gain strength and encouragement from it because your mind believes you have already done it. Get that picture in your head of The Father, the Son, and the Holy Spirit, right there, running the race with you. Nothing is impossible for God.

> Draw a picture of you with God the Father, God the Son, or the Holy Spirit. It is okay if it is stick figures and looks like a child drew it. The point is to spend time picturing what it looks like for God to physically be there with you.

ACTION

During your exercise time, think about your relationship with God the Father, God the Son, and God the Holy Spirit. Imagine them with you right now, encouraging you, cheering you on with pompons.

> Level 1: walk 1 mile as fast as you can
> Level 2: run 1-2.5 miles at your peak pace
> Level 3: run 3-7 miles at your peak pace

Turn Negatives into Positives

Scripture: Colossians 1:11-12

> May you be prepared to endure everything with patience. (Col 1:11b)

REFLECTION

You have probably heard the phrase, 'if you don't have anything nice to say, don't say anything at all.' However, not saying a negative thing about a situation or a person aloud does not mean you did not think it. This negative thought process can trip you up and keep you from seeing the goodness of God. If you get into the practice of looking for God in each situation, it can become easier to put a positive spin on things.

The scripture today is a reminder to stay strong in your words and actions to fight against negativity. This includes not only what you say but also what you think. It can be hard to change the way you think but it can be done. When terrible things happen, your mind can get stuck on the negative, but you can get unstuck with Gods help and a lot of practice.

After a while you will begin to be able to feel a difference when you say something negative verses something positive. When the negative words slip out, you might feel disappointed by your words but when you correct them or take them back, you can feel God patting you on the back, "well done my good and faithful servant" (Matt 25:23, author's paraphrase).

A disciple does not give up or give in. A disciple is prepared to endure whatever comes their way because they know God is with them. Do not let a negative thought campout inside of you because you do not have the time or energy to give to negativity. Instead, turn the negative into positive and remember to lean on God for help.

JOURNAL

As a disciple you need to think differently and that requires some work turning negative words or thoughts into positive ones. Turn your thinking around by trying to see things as half full instead of half empty. For example, when it is raining, you can be grateful you do not have to water your plants today.

Look back on the past 24-36 hours and write down negative words you have said to yourself or others. Also reflect on any negative thoughts you have had about yourself or others, these negative thoughts, though not said aloud, still effect you. After you write down the negative, try to figure out how to turn it around into something positive.

Negative word/thought you said about yourself.

How to turn the negative into a positive, what should you say instead?

Negative word/thought you said about another person.

How to turn the negative into a positive, what should you say instead?

ACTION

When you think about doing your physical or spiritual exercises each day, do you say that you *have* to or that you *get* to work on your body, mind, and spirit? The words you use can have a negative or a positive connotation. Reflect as you do your exercise on how you can focus on the positive.

Level 1: spend 15-20 minutes taking part in a cross-training activity
Level 2: spend 30-45 minutes taking part in a cross-training activity
Level 3: spend 60-90 minutes taking part in a cross-training activity

DAY 31

Be Positive

Scripture: Proverbs 3:17

> Her ways are ways of pleasantness, and all her paths
> are peace.

REFLECTION

Be positive! This is the mantra for today as you continue to work
on think more like a disciple and have a positive mindset. Positive
thinkers are pleasant to be around. They put things in a brighter
light and help lighten the load. When you meet a positive person,
you feel better about yourself just by being around them. One way
you can do to attract positivity is to think more positive thoughts
by reminding yourself with the 'be positive' mantra.

The scripture from Proverbs helps to frame this thought. When
someone is nice or pleasant to you, then you cannot help but to pass
on the good vibes. This is one reason people who volunteer say they
receive more benefit from the time they give, because they feel they
are given the opportunity to share positivity with others. Today
you will spread positivity to others with your words in the form of
a compliment. This will not only make the recipient feel good, but
you will also feel good. It is a win-win scenario.

JOURNAL

Today you are on the lookout for positivity. Your goal is to find a
positive quality or attribute for each person you encounter today,
then give them a compliment. This is how you will build the habit

of being more positive, by looking for and pointing out the positive things you see in other people. Make note of 2-3 people whom you gave a compliment, what did you say and how did they respond.

Name of the person you complimented.

Write your compliment.

What was the person's response to the compliment?

Name of the person you complimented.

Write your compliment.

What was the person's response to the compliment?

Name of the person you complimented.

Write your compliment.

What was the person's response to the compliment?

Reflect on how this activity made you feel, write down a few words to explain your experience.

ACTION

Think about the people you will compliment and what you will say. Let these images motivate you in your exercise today and possibly push you beyond what you originally planned to do.

> Level 1: take a day of rest if you need a break, it is okay to take a day off and allow your body to rejuvenate but if you are feeling good take a leisurely walk or spend 10 minutes doing a cross-training activity
> Level 2: do 15-20 minutes of yoga or stretching and 20-40 minutes of a cross-training activity
> Level 3: do 20-40 minutes of yoga or stretching and 30-60 minutes of a cross-training activity

DAY 32

New Creation

Scripture: 1 Peter 5:10

> And after you have suffered for a little while, the God of all grace, who has called you to His eternal glory in Christ, will Himself restore, support, strengthen and establish you.

REFLECTION

The scripture passage today says, God Himself will restore, support, strengthen and establish you after you have suffered. It is a reminder that God is with you always, through the good and bad. Look at Jesus' life on earth, He too faced some hardships. If anyone would have had an easy life, it would be the Son of God but instead you can look to Jesus as an example of how to endure loss and suffering.

Since there is no such thing as an easy way through life, it is guaranteed you will be challenged and tested along the way. These challenges and conflicts are necessary to go through because there are lessons you can learn about yourself and others to help you build character. They are opportunities for you to grow not only as a person but into a better disciple as well.

It is proven time after time that a person can only grow through conflict and change. You make a mistake and then you learn from it. You experience something emotionally or physically difficult, and you become a different person after going through it. You cannot expect to be the same person you were at the end of this journey as you were when you started. If you go back to your old ways, then what was all this work and sacrifice for anyway. You are being pushed and pulled and challenged through this process to come out as a new creation in Christ. Remember beauty comes from the ashes, you grow through conflict and in the process, God is refining you.

JOURNAL

Write yourself a letter to open when complete the activities in *Discipleship 5K*. In this letter to yourself, express how proud you are of the progress you have made up to this point. Put the date on your letter, seal it in an envelope and put it away until race day. It will be a gift to yourself full of encouragement and pride for all your hard work.

Dear Disciple,

ACTION

Do a bit of light stretching before and after your exercise. Remember to breathe God in with each inhale and exhale any negative feelings of stress or worry.

Level 1: walk 1-2 miles at a moderate pace
Level 2: jog 2-4 miles at a moderate pace
Level 3: run 3-7 miles at a moderate pace

WWJD – What Would Jesus Do

Scripture: Philippians 4:11

> Not that I am referring to being in need; for I have
> learned to be content with whatever I have.

REFLECTION

Whether you have nothing or if you have everything you could possibly imagine, a disciple is content with whatever they have because whatever they have is a gift from God. The life of a disciple is a series of ups and downs, but a disciple perseveres and shows gratitude for all things, in all circumstances. It is a difficult concept to grasp, especially when you are faced with a lot of exceedingly difficult life events.

Things will not always work out the way you plan but you cannot let it get you down or change your attitude from positive to negative. When you get discouraged, it takes practice to immediately put your faith and trust in God. It is easy to allow your circumstances to dictate how you feel and how you will act. However, you can make the choice to step back to allow space for prayer and reflection, so you can gain some perspective from God. Jesus did this when He needed a break or when He felt overwhelmed by the things He was doing. Remember God's ways are not your ways, and He is there ready to help you through whatever circumstance.

JOURNAL

When you experience feelings of unrest, discontentment, or are just not satisfied with a situation or a relationship, take it to prayer and ask What Would Jesus Do (WWJD)? Today, identify something in your life that you are not comfortable with, either as a part of this challenge, a situation at work, or in a personal relationship. Whatever you chose, write it down and reflect on the WWJD question. Allow time to pause and listen for a response from Jesus.

What is the situation?

What did Jesus say He would do?

ACTION

WWJD. Today put forth the effort Jesus would as you take part in your cross-training activity.

Levèl 1: spend at least 15 minutes doing a cross-training activity

Level 2: spend at least 30 minutes doing a cross-training activity

Level 3: spend at least 60 minutes doing a cross-training activity

DAY 34

Check Yourself

Scripture: Ecclesiastes 7:9

> Do not be quick to anger, for anger lodges in the
> bosom of fools.

REFLECTION

As you become more disciplined in your faith, the devil will take notice and begin to put obstacles in your way. He will do whatever is necessary to keep you from looking for and having a deeper relationship with God. Perhaps you have already experienced the devil trying to distract you from reaching your goal of becoming a better disciple.

You cannot battle the devil on your own, you are human and will fall victim to sin and at times will let your negative emotions lead your actions. It is normal to let responsibilities and the demands of the world get the best of you. Everyone has tried to fit one more thing into an already busy schedule and become frustrated when things do not work out as planned. It is okay to get overwhelmed, but you do not want to have any innocent victims hurt in your wrath.

When temptation gets the best of you, and you find yourself lashing out, it is best to apologize right away. Do not allow pride to get in the way of an apology or give you an excuse for behaving badly. When you are working on being a better person, you will need to take responsibility for your emotions and actions. The more disciplined you become, the less the devil will bother you because he will get the message you do not have room in your life for his silly distractions.

JOURNAL

It is time to apologize to someone you have hurt. Perhaps it was because you were grouchy, tired, or upset due to work stress, relationship stress, financial stress or a million other things. Do not allow your frustrations or stress to be hurtful to others, there is never a good reason to lash out on someone. Today, apologize and take responsibility for your actions.

> Write an apology note here to practice what you will say to this person whom you have wronged in some way. Then go apologize.

ACTION

Do some light stretching before and after your walk. Practice deep breathing while you reflect on your transgressions.

> Level 1: take a 1.5-3-mile leisurely walk
> Level 2: take a 2–4-mile leisurely walk or jog
> Level 3: take a 4–6-mile leisurely jog

DAY 35

No Shortcuts

Scripture: Luke 6:37-38

> For the measure you give will be the measure you get back. (Luke 6:38b)

REFLECTION

Time is an important commodity. It seems there is never enough time to do everything you want to do. Where does the time go? You might have complained before that you did not have time to pray or spend time with God. Perhaps in the past you neglected God, even when you were given opportunities to spend time with Him.

You get out what you put in. This statement is true of everything, and the scripture spells it out perfectly. If you spend 30 minutes preparing a home cooked meal, it is going to be healthier than spending the same time waiting for a pizza to be delivered. When you take shortcuts, you do not get to reap the complete reward. It is the same with the time you give to God. The more time you give in prayer or service to others, the more God will open up time for you.

God calls his disciples to love Him and to love others. So, when you slow down and lend a hand to your neighbor even though you are running late for an appointment, many times, God somehow helps you reach your destination on time. It is quite amazing to see God show up in that way and He does it when you least expect it.

Reflect on how you divide your time in a normal week. Do you spend your time doing things that reflect your beliefs and what you consider important? If not, it is time to reprioritize so you can be a better disciple. As a disciple you should reflect God's love.

Consider ways you already do this and brainstorm ways you could do this in the future. A terrific way to reflect God's love is by volunteering or doing something of service for someone in need. It does not need to take a lot of time, for example, you might volunteer to take a meal to someone who is undergoing chemotherapy, or you might mow your neighbor's yard because they just brought home a newborn. There are no shortcuts to discipleship, but God can reward you with the time you need to do what He calls you to do if you let Him.

JOURNAL

Make time to volunteer your time by helping someone close to you who is in need or going out into your community to give time. Allow God to be the keeper of your time and volunteer to do something extra soon.

> Write down five different volunteer opportunities available to you right now.

ACTION

Imagine the different ways you can give your time to others while you do your activity today.

Level 1: practice 15-20 minutes of yoga or stretching
and do 15-20 minutes of a cross-training activity
Level 2: practice 20-30 minutes of yoga or stretching
and do 30-60 minutes of a cross-training activity
Level 3: practice 30-60 minutes of yoga or stretching
and do 45-60 minutes of a cross-training activity

WEEK FIVE OVERVIEW

Write down any thoughts, words of encouragement, ideas for growth or measurements of progress you have from this week from your physical and spiritual training.

WEEK SIX
Inspiration from the World

This week marks the halfway point of *Discipleship 5K*, and you might be teeter-tottering between the good and the bad of the challenge. It is time to go in search of some words of wisdom to help get you over the hump and keep you moving forward towards your goal. You do not only get inspiration from the Bible, but from people all over the world. Your hard work is paying off, you have come so far but you are not in this alone. There are several people who are known for being motivational speakers or having said something inspirational and their words are there to remind you how formidable you are for all you have done and to encourage you to do more.

For example, Oprah Winfrey said, "Life is about growth and change." These words are great for this challenge because you can look back at how you have grown and changed through the process. You can use your journal entries to remind you of how far you have come since the beginning and help you identify some changes you still want to make. It is a reminder that life is not about standing still but about forming and reforming yourself into the person you and God want you to be.

DAY 36

You Came - You Saw - You Conquered

Scripture: Proverbs 24:32

> Then I saw and considered it; I looked and received
> instruction.

REFLECTION

When you began this training, it might have been the first time
you ever committed to walking or running in a 5K or, it might have
been the first time you read scripture from the Bible. It could be the
first time you made a commitment to spend time working on being
a better follower of Christ. Even if it was not the first time for you
to do any of these things, it was still a change of behavior from your
normal, everyday actions. You began something new.

At the start of any new task, it takes a while to train yourself
to talk differently and act differently to be successful. When you
made the commitment to become a better disciple, it required you
to learn some new skills, it demanded you live your life with more
intention, more purpose. These physical and spiritual exercises have
been guiding you on this journey. You deserve a pat on the back for
all your arduous work to get you to this halfway point.

You came. You saw. You conquered. These words are another
way of saying what the author of Proverbs is saying in the scripture.
They are a reminder of how hard you have been working and how
proud you should be for all you have accomplished. Even though
there is still half the challenge ahead of you, there is no reason you
cannot celebrate, so long as you do not forget the reward that awaits
you as you continue to grow closer to God. It will definitely be
worth it!

JOURNAL

Make a list of the things you have learned so far on this journey about yourself, about others and about God. Also make a note of your favorite physical activities and spiritual activities. These reflections will be motivators when you look back over the challenge to remind you of the progress you have made along the way.

What you have learned about yourself.

What you have learned about others.

What you have learned about God.

What are your favorite physical activities?

What are your favorite spiritual activities?

Now that you are halfway through the training you might need to change things up a little bit. Try a new activity on your cross-training days or add a new daily prayer to your regimen; something new and different to help you stay on the path to success on this journey. Make a note about what you will change.

NEW Physical Activity

NEW Spiritual Activity

ACTION

Take time before and after your exercise to stretch.

Level 1: walk 1-2 miles at a moderate pace
Level 2: jog 2-4 miles at a moderate pace
Level 3: run 3-7 miles at a moderate pace

DAY 37

Press On

Scripture: Philippians 3:12-16

I press on toward the goal. (Phil 3:14)

REFLECTION

It takes a lot of discipline to stay true to a goal. There are rules you must follow and sometimes you must resist doing things that will keep you from reaching your goal. When you make a commitment to achieve a goal, you must stay dedicated to the goal. It is true of any type of commitment you make whether you are committed to training for a 5K or if your goal is to be a disciple.

Goals are not achieved with one big swoop; they are achieved little by little. It is a good reminder at this point in the challenge. In the pursuit of any goal there will be obstacles you will face, and you must figure out how you will rise above. Remember that those obstacles are there to teach you and make you stronger. Now is not the time to grow complacent. At this point, there is even more need to stay persistent, work to keep it interesting and continue to grow both physically and spiritually.

JOURNAL

Today the reflection asks you to create an action plan with specific steps you will take to achieve your goal. Create action steps, specific things you will do to achieve the goal. It might be three steps or five steps or more. Write out whatever it will take for you to stay on track.

Identify your action steps for physical progress.

Identify your action steps for spiritual progress.

ACTION

While you stretch, reflect on the journal question. Call on God to help you identify your action steps.

> Level 1: spend 15-20 minutes doing yoga or stretching and 15-20 minutes taking part in a cross-training activity
> Level 2: spend 20-40 minutes doing yoga or stretching and 20-40 minutes taking part in a cross-training activity
> Level 3: spend 30-60 minutes doing yoga or stretching and 30-60 minutes taking part in a cross-training activity

DAY 38

One Body of Christ

Scripture: Galatians 3:28

> There is no longer Jew or Greek, there is no longer slave or free, there is no longer male and female; for all of you are one in Christ Jesus.

REFLECTION

These words of scripture from Saint Paul to the Galatians are a reminder to you of how God is with you and makes you whole through baptism. And how through your Baptism you were born into a new family where everyone is one in Christ Jesus. This means you have many brothers and sisters in Christ and are not alone, ever.

You are not alone on this physical and spiritual journey either. As a member of the *Discipleship 5K* community, you have others doing the same challenges and completing the same reflections. You are also not the only one who will take part in a 5K race. There will be many people walking, running, or cheering friends and family members on as they compete.

It is nice to have others to lean on for support and know you are not alone in this experience. This is what being a disciple is all about, the community of believers who support one another. If you have not already found the *Discipleship 5K* community on the *Making Scripture Relevant* Facebook page or subscribed to watch the daily reflection for *Discipleship 5K* on YouTube, it is not too late. These resources are there to encourage you and for you to know there are others out there doing the same work.

JOURNAL

During a real 5K race, there are people along the race path with signs and pom-poms who cheer on the participants and wait for them at the finish line. Have you invited others to take part in the 5K with you? Who will come to cheer you on? Today, shout out to those people who are cheering you on by making a list of people who have been encouraging you since you started the challenge. Make a point to invite them to come and support you on the day of the race.

If you are going to take part in an actual race, it is time to research and sign up. If you decide this is not your final goal, start planning a fun event for yourself so those who have been encouraging you along the way can come cheer you on and celebrate all your hard work.

> Write the names of the people who have been encouraging you along the way.

ACTION

Invite one of the people who have been encouraging you to join you in your cross-training activity today.

> Level 1: spend at least 30 minutes taking part in a cross-training activity
> Level 2: spend at least 45 minutes taking part in a cross-training activity
> Level 3: spend at least 60 minutes taking part in a cross-training activity

DAY 39

Stand Strong

Scripture: Acts 5:27-29

> Peter and the apostles answered, "We must obey
> God rather than any human authority." (Acts 5:29)

REFLECTION

You are given tests each day, in everyday circumstances when you must decide to move forward or to stand still. Some decisions are fairly easy, and sometimes you may not even know a decision was made, such as whether you will have cereal or toast for breakfast. Other decisions require thought and effort such as, will you resist walking by the snack machine and stopping for a treat or will you eat the carrots and hummus you brought from home.

There are millions of decisions you must make each day, and each of them are opportunities for you to do the right thing and live more intentionally as a disciple. God gave you freewill so that you would decide to choose Him. The decisions you make throughout the day are practice for you so when faced with the decision, you will already know what to decide. Look to the Disciples in the scripture as an example of how to stand up for what you believe and do what is right.

Yesterday you focused on the people who have been supportive on this journey but not everyone is going to be supportive of you taking part in the activities set out for you in *Discipleship 5K*. There may be some who are jealous of you or do not understand why you would do something like this. Others might be upset because you used to spend more time with them and now you are too busy working exercising and praying.

When you say *yes* to one thing, you are saying *no* to something else. This can be a challenge for some people to accept. However, there is nothing wrong with deciding to focus on your physical and spiritual health. Be strong in what you believe is right.

JOURNAL

Take a little time to find your core values and create a personal mission statement. These will be the things you will stand up for and fight to keep. If you are not familiar with mission statements, spend time researching mission statements on the internet. Every company has a mission statement for the business, the employees and potential customers which broadcasts the values the company stands for and the goal or goals of the company.

Brainstorm ten attributes you believe important (i.e., trust, strength, integrity).

Then trim the list down to a top three.

Use these three words to create a personal mission statement for your life.

ACTION

Be sure you are making the time to do some light stretching before and after you do your exercise. Do not rush through the stretching because it is an important piece of taking care of your body.

Level 1: walk 1-2 miles at a moderate pace
Level 2: jog 2-4 miles at a moderate pace
Level 3: run 3-7 miles at a moderate pace

The Cross

Scripture: Ecclesiastes 3:17

> I said in my heart, God will judge the righteous and
> the wicked, for he has appointed a time for every
> matter, and for every work.

REFLECTION

There is nothing too difficult for you to overcome. Whenever you
think something is hard or if you are too tired to do your exercise,
reflect on the cross of Jesus. He endured so much more than you
will ever have to, so be encouraged by this knowledge, and use it to
help you to persevere. You made a commitment to dedicate time to
yourself and to God and become more fit, physically, and spiritually.

At times it probably seems like it would be easier if you would
just throw in the towel and forget you ever started. This is all a part
of the process. When you made the decision to follow Jesus, you said
'yes' to walking the road to Calvary with Him. You will experience
times of feeling beaten, you will want to give up, you will fall down,
and you will at times want to quit. However, when you compare
what Jesus suffered, with what you are dealing with right now, it
may not seem so bad. And like Jesus, after the suffering, there is
resurrection, so keep going, the victory is coming.

JOURNAL

Spend time meditating on the cross. Think about the struggles
Jesus endured and the great victory that is still celebrated today.

Reflect on any struggles you have right now and write them down. After you have identified them, imagine laying them at the foot of the cross and handing them over to Jesus. This action can be helpful in removing any obstacles in your path, such as negative thoughts or unrealistic expectations that might be distracting you from completing your daily physical and spiritual exercises.

> Write down the struggles you want to lie at the foot
> of the cross.

ACTION

Make sure you are stretching before and after you exercises to help prevent injury.

> Level 1: participate in 10-15 minutes of a cross-training activity and do 10-15 minutes of a weight training activity
> Level 2: participate in 20-30 minutes of a cross-training activity and do 10-15 minutes of a weight training activity
> Level 3: participate in 45-60 minutes of a cross-training activity and do 15-20 minutes of a weight training activity

DAY 41

Not Alone

Scripture: Psalm 10:17-18

> O Lord, you will hear the desire of the meek.
> (Ps 10:17a)

REFLECTION

As you dedicate yourself more deeply to the new habits of prayer and physical activity, the devil will tempt you. He will sprinkle doubt in your mind. You might think you do not have time to pray or to do your reflection or workout. There will be obstacles that pop-up and begin to weigh on you.

It is easy to get down and become distracted. This challenge takes twelve weeks because you need to train your body and your mind so it is strong enough to overcome the obstacles the devil will throw at you. So, when you feel like you are being singled out and attacked from all angles, remember you are not alone. Your inclination will be to quit or slow down because those negatives are easy to believe but you cannot forget there are many others on this journey with you.

One of the best ways to overcome the obstacles you face is to find companions who can support you and whom you can give encouragement to as well. When you walk with others, you become stronger because you know you are not alone. You have someone talk to when you are discouraged, who will understand your struggles. It is nice to hear encouraging words, but it is just as nice to say them to others. You were not called to run this race alone; rather you are called to be there for one another.

JOURNAL

Jesus had companions on His walk to Calvary. There were those who helped carry the cross, others to wipe His face and still others who were there to encourage Him. You have companions too; you just need to take time to identify them.

Find someone you know who is taking part in a 5K race or who you know has recently started a new routine. Ask them how they are doing and if they are making progress. It is nice to be able to connect with another person who is going through what you are going through, or at least something similar. Their experience can give you possible insight on your own journey or simply help you feel like you have someone you can talk to about what you are learning through the process. You might even find you are not the one who needs the pick me up and instead you become the encourager.

> Write about the experience of reaching out to someone. Who did you contact and what came about from the conversation?

ACTION

Practice your breathing for at least five minutes and stretch before and after your exercise. If your body needs a rest day, today would be a good day to take a break from your physical activity and focus on the journal exercise.

Level 1: take a 1.5-3-mile leisurely walk
Level 2: take a 2–4-mile leisurely walk or jog
Level 3: take a 4–6-mile leisurely jog

DAY 42

Rest in Him

Scripture: John 14:1-14

> Do not let your hearts be troubled. Believe in God,
> believe also in me. (John 14:1)

REFLECTION

The scripture passage for today is a reminder that when you believe in God, you also believe in Jesus. When you add the Spirit, you have the Holy Trinity. Think of the body, mind, and spirit connection as the Holy Trinity of self-care. Just as God, Jesus and the Holy Spirit are one, you need to work on all three elements of your personal health to find peace.

There are times when you can feel discouraged, especially when things do not go the way you think they should go. This feeling can take over and cause you to lose sight of the task at hand. There is nothing the devil wants more than for you to trip up and get off balance. When you fall victim to the devil's tricks, remind yourself that you belong to God; body, mind, and spirit to help you get back on track.

God made you in His image and likeness. This does not mean God looks like you, though He sent his son Jesus to earth as a human. Instead, God breathed into you so that your soul, your spirit is like God. It is time to use that power for good and squash any distractions the devil has put in your path. Take time to rest in Him today through your yoga and stretching so you can connect God and your spirit together to find the peace He wants you to have in your life.

JOURNAL

Take out your Bible and ask God to lead you to the words you need to hear today. Choose a random piece of scripture to meditate on while you stretch. Perhaps, use your birthday month and day as the chapter and verse of the scripture. Whatever piece of scripture you choose, it is time to rest in God and allow the words to soak into your soul.

> Write down the scripture you turned to and spend time in quiet reflection.

> What did God say to you through the scripture verse you reflected on?

ACTION

Think about the mind, body, spirit connection while you practice your yoga or stretching.

> Level 1: practice 15-20 minutes of yoga or stretching and do 15-20 minutes of a cross-training activity
> Level 2: practice 20-30 minutes of yoga or stretching and do 30-60 minutes of a cross-training activity
> Level 3: practice 30-60 minutes of yoga or stretching and do 45-60 minutes of a cross-training activity

WEEK SIX OVERVIEW

Write down any thoughts, words of encouragement, ideas for growth or measurements of progress you have from this week from your physical and spiritual training.

WEEK SEVEN
Motivation from the Communion of Saints

Last week you looked for motivational quotes from people who inspire you. This week, find encouragement from the lives of the Saints, people who lived out their discipleship imperfectly. You are bound to find much comfort and strength from the Saints. Plus, their life stories can help you understand how God works in and through those He loves.

This week as you dive into the lives of the Saints, remember they are people who made it to the cross. Their stories are notable examples of what it takes to be a disciple and to follow God. The scripture each day will give examples of how changing your mindset can help you more easily recognize God's presence in your life. Embrace the encouragement because there is still plenty of work to do; hills to climb, figuratively and literally. Turning to the Communion of Saints and those in the *Discipleship 5K* community are great tools to help get you through this week and beyond.

DAY 43

Special Gifts

Scripture: 1 Corinthians 12:4-31

> To each is given the manifestation of the Spirit for the common good. (1 Cor 12:7)

REFLECTION

The scripture today is a reminder that God's desire is not for each person to be a clone of one another. Instead, He created everyone with their own likes and dislikes, their own special gifts. God desires everyone to use the unique gifts they have to honor Him by working together to compliment and support one another.

So, it is time to recognize those extraordinary gifts in others and encourage them. You do this by identifying a unique skill or a special talent of another person, and then telling them that you appreciate it. Everyone deserves an attagirl or attaboy so they know they are something special. When you honor the gifts of others, you can also gain understanding in how their gifts and talents compliment your own. Acknowledging their gifts can also highlight some of your own that you did not know you had.

JOURNAL

Encourage another person today, share a positive word with another person, acknowledge a job well done or simply let them know how much they mean to you. Your positive words will remind them of the personal gifts God has given them and inspire them to continue to share their God given gifts with others.

You do not have to do it in person either. Write a note or an email. Give someone a call. Regardless of how you choose to reach out, everyone loves to hear they are doing something good and that they are being noticed.

Who did you encourage?

What is their special gift?

What words did you use to compliment them?

How did they respond to your compliment?

How do their special gifts compliment your own gifts?

ACTION

Reflect on the encouraging words you said to another person and use them on yourself to push you during your exercise today. If you are taking part in a cross-training class, encourage at least one person in the class whom you have never met, in addition to the journal exercise. There is no limit to the number of people you can encourage today or any other day.

> Level 1: participate in at least 30 minutes of a cross-training activity
> Level 2: participate in at least 45 minutes of a cross-training activity
> Level 3: participate in at least 60 minutes of a cross-training activity

Cheerful Heart

Scripture: Proverbs 15:13-15

A cheerful heart has a continual feast. (Prov 15:15b)

REFLECTION

The scripture says to have a cheerful heart because a sorrowful heart is a broken heart. It is scientifically proven that it takes more muscles to frown than it does to smile. There are also scientific studies that show that you can raise your dopamine and serotonin levels (chemicals that increase happiness) when you act happy, even if you do not feel happy. This means you should smile more because it is good for your physical and emotional health.

It is also said that 'laughter is the best medicine' which means you should laugh regularly to help you feel better. Sometimes when you are working toward a goal, you get so focused on the goal, and you forget to have some fun. Though becoming a better disciple is serious business, you do not need to be so serious that you forget to have fun and laugh. You might even find the occasion to laugh at yourself if you allow yourself to relax a bit.

JOURNAL

Are you having fun yet? Scientific studies have proven it is good for your health to go out and do something fun, laugh a little or a lot and try to make it a regular habit. Do not keep the fun to yourself, call a friend or multiple friends and make plans to do something together. They might be looking for a way to have a more cheerful heart too.

Write down what you will do today or very soon to have some fun.

ACTION

Start your exercise time out with a laugh by looking at yourself in the mirror and making a silly face. Also do 5-10 minutes of calisthenics before and after your walk or run.

> Level 1: walk 1 mile as fast as you can
> Level 2: run 1-2.5 miles at your peak pace
> Level 3: run 3-7 miles at your peak pace

DAY 45

Give God Credit

Scripture: 2 Corinthians 4:5-10

> So that it may be made clear that this extraordinary power belongs to God and does not come from us. (2 Cor 4:7b)

REFLECTION

Making God a priority in your life is not always easy. However, it is easy to get in the habit of putting your own needs above the needs of others and of God. When you put your needs above others, your actions are saying you do not really care too much about the needs of another. This means God too.

To follow God means you follow the commandments. It can be difficult at times, especially putting God first because He is not physically there nagging or reminding you that He wants your attention. Plus, the world is constantly in your face with messages that tell you to do it your way; and life is all about you and to do whatever makes you happy.

In the scripture passage today, Saint Paul's Letter to the Corinthians is a great reminder to not get boastful or let your ego take credit for the good you do. Instead, give God the credit. At this point in the challenge, you have made some great strides and accomplished a lot, but you cannot forget to express gratitude to God for being there with you every step of the way. It is time to acknowledge God for all He does and has done. Make sure you have time in your schedule specifically for God. You know He deserves it.

JOURNAL

Find the Ten Commandments in your Bible, Exodus 20:2-17. Think about how you have lived each of those out this past week by putting God and others before yourself.

> On a scale from 1-10, how well do you feel you are following the Ten Commandments?

> Focus on the first three commandments which pertain to your relationship with God.
> How did you uphold these commandments this week? Name specific ways you followed them.

> Write down ways you did not follow the first three commandments. What adjustments can you make to be more successful next week. Be specific.

Focus on the last seven commandments which pertain to your relationship with others.

How did you uphold these commandments this past week? Name specific ways you followed them.

Write down ways you did not follow the last seven commandments. What adjustments can you make to be more successful next week. Be specific.

Do you think the first three commandments are easier or harder to follow than the last seven? Explain.

Write a prayer asking God to help you to be more mindful of Him and others next week.

ACTION

Practice breathing deeply either during your exercise time or outside of it to reflect on the Ten Commandments. Each time you draw in a breath, think of one of the commandments, hold your breath and then as you exhale ask God to help you keep that commandment.

Level 1: spend 15-20 minutes doing yoga or stretching and take part in 15-20 minutes of a cross-training activity

Level 2: spend 20-40 minutes doing yoga or stretching and take part in 20-40 minutes of a cross-training activity

Level 3: spend 30-60 minutes doing yoga or stretching and take part in 30-60 minutes of a cross-training activity

Be Yourself

Scripture: 2 Timothy 3:10-17

> But as for you, continue in what you have learned and firmly believed, knowing from whom you learned it. (2 Tim 3:14)

REFLECTION

It is a popular plotline in movies, books and plays for a character to try to be something they are not by changing their hair color, their clothes, and their behavior. Sometimes this is done for the purpose of hiding their own identity to achieve a goal such as a female disguising herself as a male so she can play on a specific sports team. Other times they hide their identity for protection from harm or so they can cause it. Still other times they do it to learn a different perspective as in the stories where characters trade lives and try to be the other person. In every scenario the deception cannot last.

God did not create you to be something or someone you are not; He wants you to be you. When you try to be anything other than your true self, you are not being genuine. And to use the words of the scripture passage, "imposters will go from bad to worse, deceiving others and being deceived" (2 Tim 3:13). Making it clear that nothing good can come from trying to be something you are not. A disciple strives to be the person God created them to be and that means doing everything you can to be the best version of yourself. It does not mean you try to be someone else, just be you.

JOURNAL

It can be a major struggle in life, trying to figure out what you want to be when you grow up and what you want to achieve in your life. However, when you look at yourself the way God sees you, it is easy to decipher that you are called to be a disciple. So, what are the traits of a disciple and do you have them? Today you will find out. Spend time reflecting on the traits of a disciple and use the Bible to help you make the list.

> What are the qualities a disciple should have according to the Bible?

> Write down one or two traits of a disciple that you want to build up in your life.

ACTION

Choose one of the traits to reflect on while you do your exercise and try to put it into action.

> Level 1: participate in 10-15 minutes of a cross-training activity and spend 10-15 minutes doing a weight training activity
>
> Level 2: participate in 20-30 minutes of a cross-training activity and spend 10-15 minutes doing a weight training activity
>
> Level 3: participate in 60-90 minutes of a cross-training activity and spend 15-20 minutes doing a weight training activity

DAY 47

Role Models

Scripture: Leviticus chapters 19-20

> You shall be holy, for I the Lord your God am holy.
> (Lev 19:2)

REFLECTION

The scripture today is Leviticus chapters 19 and 20; chapter 19 is God's list of qualities a person should practice or live out and chapter 20 is the list of things they should not. This scripture from Leviticus came to before on this journey of *Discipleship 5k* on Day 3 and is back again so you can reflect on how you have changed to become more of the person God wants you to be.

God calls you to be yourself and since you are made "in His image" (Gen 1:27), you are holy as He is holy. So, as you grow in your discipleship, you reflect more and more of God's holiness. You can learn good traits by spending time in prayer and through the study of Scripture, and by answering the call to treat God and others with love and respect.

Yes, there will be times when you do not treat others the way you should. You might get caught up in the wrong crowd doing the wrong things which can take you further and further away from God. However, through the exercises of *Discipleship 5K*, you are learning how to instill good habits in your life to help you to become more holy. God sent Jesus to be a living example, a role model of how to be holy.

JOURNAL

Yesterday you made a list of traits you believe a disciple should have and now it is time to check in to see how you are living it out these traits in your life. You also want to think about people in your life who have the traits of a disciple and are using their special gifts to reflect God's holiness. Perhaps those people who are living the faith and being genuine can serve as role models to you.

Think about people in your life who have the qualities of a disciple, someone who is reflecting God's holiness. These people can be alive or dead, as long as it is someone you can look at and say they lived or are living a genuine life. This is your list of role models who will be there to encourage you through this challenge and in life.

Role Model #1

What traits does this person have that you want to emulate?

Role Model #2

What traits does this person have that you want to emulate?

Role Model #3

What traits does this person have that you want to emulate?

Role Model #4

What traits does this person have that you want to emulate?

Role Model #5

What traits does this person have that you want to emulate?

Write a prayer to God asking for help to be more like the role models you have chosen so you can learn to be more Holy like Him.

ACTION

As you practice your breathing, think of how you will weave holiness into your daily practices. Do not forget to stretch before and after your exercise; it will give you more time to reflect on holiness.

> Level 1: walk 1-2 miles at a moderate pace
> Level 2: jog 2-4 miles at a moderate pace
> Level 3: run 3-7 miles at a moderate pace

DAY 48

Share Love

Scripture: 1 Corinthians 13:4-7

> It [love] bears all things, believes all things, hopes
> all things, endures all things. (1 Cor 13:7)

REFLECTION

Today's scripture comes from 1 Corinthians, chapter 13. It is the love scripture, often read at weddings. It explains what love is and what love is not.

It is often said that God is love so you can read the scripture replacing the word love with God. You can go even further and say your name in place of the word love. When you read it aloud, it can be a spiritual experience. You can even write the scripture out with your name replacing the word love so you can see it and use it as a reminder when you forget.

This exercise can help open your body, mind, and spirit in a new way. It can remind you of who God calls you to be and how He wants you to show up for Him and others. You are called to be true and honest with yourself and with others. These words of scripture are one of God's little reminders to find joy in doing good for others and to be love to one another.

JOURNAL

It is time to show love differently by doing something for someone that you do not want to do. This is a way to let them know you love them and do it without expecting something in return.

To whom will you show love?

What will you do to show love?

Additionally, make two columns of what love is and what love is not according to the scripture.

Love Is   Love Is Not

ACTION

Reflect on the word LOVE while you stretch before and after your exercise.

Level 1: take a 2–4-mile leisurely walk
Level 2: take a 3–5-mile leisurely walk or jog
Level 3: take a 5–7-mile leisurely jog

Forgive Yourself

Scripture: Mark 2:21

> No one sews a piece of unshrunk cloth on an old cloak, otherwise, the patch pulls away from it, the new from the old and a worse tear is made.

REFLECTION

The scripture says you cannot patch an old coat with a new patch, it just does not work. When you drink out of a paper cup, it can only be used a few times before it begins to collapse. There are things in your life that are like the paper cup, you have used it for its purpose and now it is time to get rid of it. You might have some old shoes getting in your way and cluttering your closet, perhaps there are some old coats which are too small for you taking up space too. We need to get rid of the old things and make room for the new. This does not only apply for things in your house, but this can also be done with old thoughts or feelings that weigh you down.

Through this challenge you have been making new habits for your physical and spiritual health and you cannot go back to your old ways or fall into the immoral behavior patterns. God is working on you to become a new creation. The old habits no longer have the same effect or meaning.

This is the new you, the one who allows for a hiccup or two. The person who can and will let go of small stresses and does not let little hurts fester into big ones. You are stronger than you were when you began. You are different because you are being intentional about being a better disciple. This does not mean you are perfect or that you always do everything that is expected of you. It does mean you are more aware of the way God sees things and you more willingly accept grace when it is needed.

Today let go of any guilt or frustration you hold within this challenge. Anything that is causing you to feel like you are not doing enough; forgive yourself and allow yourself some grace. Stop counting the days when you walked instead of ran or when you skipped a workout all together. God is not keeping a timer on the amount of time you spend in prayer so you should not either. It is time to refresh, restart and renew. You get to start over, regardless of any days you have missed a reflection or did not read the scripture. Start over. Hit the refresh button and let go of anything that is holding you back. Jesus is waiting for you at the finish line.

JOURNAL

Make of list of reasons you cannot or should not finish this training commitment. Do these thoughts get in your way of doing your best? For each item on the list, write something you will do to overcome that obstacle. For example, if one of the reasons you are not training as you ought to be is because it is too hot or cold outside, make a point to work out at a different time of the day, rearrange your schedule to accommodate. Or, if you are several days behind on your scripture, reflection and actions just begin with the actual day you are on and let go of the days you have missed. Think of it as if you are just starting over fresh and new. Let go and shed the excuses so you can begin again.

Obstacle

Plan to overcome

Obstacle

Plan to overcome

Obstacle

Plan to overcome

ACTION

Listen to your body and do what is best for you. Remember these are suggestions and guidelines; do not let them be an obstacle in your path to get to the finish line.

> Level 1: practice 15-20 minutes of yoga or stretching and take part in 20-30 minutes of a cross-training activity
> Level 2: practice 20-30 minutes of yoga or stretching and take part in 30-60 minutes of a cross-training activity
> Level 3: practice 30-60 minutes of yoga or stretching and take part in 45-60 minutes of a cross-training activity

WEEK SEVEN OVERVIEW

Write down any thoughts, words of encouragement, ideas for growth or measurements of progress you have from this week from your physical and spiritual training.

WEEK EIGHT
Role Models of Faith

Jesus understood, maybe more than anyone that the road to the cross requires hard work and suffering. This is the lesson He was trying to teach when He said, "Enter through the narrow gate; for the gate is wide and the road is easy that leads to destruction, and there are many who take it. For the gate is narrow and the road is hard that leads to life, and there are few who find it" (Matt 7:14). And when He told a Rich Young Man that, "it is easier for a camel to go through the eye of a needle than for someone who is rich to enter the kingdom of God" (Matt 19:16-30). Jesus wanted everyone to understand that to follow God's Law and live the life of a disciple meant making sacrifices and sometimes doing things that are against popular opinion.

The good news about this lesson is, Jesus did not just preach this lifestyle, He lived it. And through living it, Jesus became the number one role model of how to live it. So, today you might feel worn out, tired and beat up but you are so close to completing the second month of *Discipleship 5K*. Do not discount the good you have done, nor the blood, sweat and tears you have lost along the way. Remember to lean on Jesus when you begin to feel like the road is too hard; Jesus has been there and conquered that already!

Pope Francis said, "To be a Saint is not a privilege for a few but a vocation for everyone." This week, look to the saints for encouragement as you make the changes you need to be successful through to the end. Saints are examples; good role models to follow especially when you learn about the hard things they lived through and how they endured pain or suffered while still putting God first.

You are a saint in training. You do not have to be Catholic to find inspiration from a saint. They are just like any friend or family member who has died, and you can spend time learning about or looking back on their lives. Take time to research if there is a saint who shares your first name or middle name; perhaps even your birthday. Read about their lives and see if you have anything in common with them. You could even find a patron saint of something that interests you. Believe it or not there are patron saints for needleworkers, athletes, mothers and just about everything. There is nothing to lose and a new friend to gain. Go be inspired.

DAY 50
Keep Fighting
Scripture: Judges chapter 4

> If you go with me, I will go. If you do not go with
> me, I will not go. (Judg 4:8)

REFLECTION

God says repeatedly in the Scripture that He is with you always. Whenever you turn from God, God remains faithful. It is a hard lesson to learn because life is a series of ups and downs. Sometimes you are doing great and other times you find yourself feeling like there is no end to the pain or suffering. There is no real consistency, except that God is there even if He feels a million miles away. Even when you feel like you are fighting a battle all alone, you need to trust God is there.

Reflect on some of the battles you have faced in your life. You might have fought a few or several. Some might be external and others internal. Even in this challenge, you could have faced a battle with time or between your mind and your body. However, you have made it here to Day 50 which means you are strong. Keep fighting to find the time to exercise and to pray. Call on God to be with you in this battle. He will bring his Son; Jesus and His secret weapon the Holy Spirit to fight alongside you. They have won the victory *for* you, now it is time to win it *with* you.

JOURNAL

Today in your prayer, invite God into your struggle. He is there for you and might have some friends who can relate to what you are going through. You do not need to trudge through the muck alone. Like the Beatles said, "you can get by with a little help from your friends." When you are in relationship with God, you will more readily recognize the people whom God gives you to bring comfort or kindness or even companionship. As you continue the work necessary to grow and deepen your relationship with God, you need to be more aware of His presence. If God is always with you, then you should see Him.

> Write a prayer acknowledging God's presence and invite Him to join you in it.

> Search for God in your training today. Where did you find Him?

ACTION

Spend at least 5 minutes practicing breathing deeply. Try breathing in through your nose, count to seven and then hold the breath for five counts and slowly breathe out your nose.

Level 1: spend 10-15 minutes doing a cross-training activity and 10-15 minutes doing a weight training activity

Level 2: spend 20-30 minutes doing a cross-training activity and 10-15 minutes doing a weight training activity

Level 3: spend 60-90 minutes doing a cross-training activity and 15-20 minutes doing a weight training activity

God is Your Refuge

Scripture: Psalm 46:1

> God is our refuge and strength, a very present help
> in trouble.

REFLECTION

Sometimes the mountain you are trying to climb seems so overwhelming that you cannot fathom how you will get over it. It can be frustrating when you continue to hit roadblocks or have obstacles on the path. When you feel down or discouraged, it affects not only your own attitude but others around you too. It can be exceedingly difficult to get yourself out of a funky mood or to begin to feel better, especially after something negative happens. It is a battle.

There will be moments when you feel deflated because you think you should be further along. Maybe you are doing the best you can and giving your all, but the results you desire are still out of reach. It is only natural to feel disappointed, but your attitude makes all the difference. When your heart is not in it, you can tell because you are not able to finish strong, or maybe even start at all.

You want to be able to look back and say you did your best. Many professional athletes use this tactic, often called the 'leave it all on the field' mentality which means you give everything you have, so regardless of the outcome, you will have no regrets knowing you did all you could to succeed. This mindset can work for you too when you are feeling deflated from all life is throwing at you. It most certainly applies to the level of effort you put towards your prayer and your workout activities prescribed in *Discipleship 5K*.

The mindset of a disciple is to persevere because you know God is your refuge and strength. This fact is confirmed in scripture, and not just in the passage you read today. Throughout the Bible there are stories of how God shows up to heal and bring comfort to His people. He walks through the grim times with them, and He gives them the power to overcome.

The verse from Psalms today does not just say God is your refuge and strength, but that He is a very present help in your times of trouble. It is such great news to know God is there even when you do not acknowledge Him. He is just waiting for you to turn your struggle or conflict over to Him. God is ready to show up for you 100% and take each step with you. Turn to God in the scripture and seek His words of encouragement, words that make you feel strong and capable. When you bring God into the struggle, you are more likely able to get through it; disciples know this, and they live it.

JOURNAL

God's Word, the scripture, is full of encouraging passages, ones that remind you of your strength and how you can do all things. Turn to the words of scripture and let them become your fight song as you tackle these next few weeks. Find, write down and memorize three scripture verses to help encourage yourself on this journey.

Scripture Verse #1

Scripture Verse #2

Scripture Verse #3

ACTION

Before and after your exercise to do 5-10 minutes of calisthenics and remember not to rush your stretching.

Level 1: walk 1.5 miles as fast as you can
Level 2: run 1.5-3 miles at your peak pace
Level 3: run 4-8 miles at your peak pace

Find Joy

Scripture: Job 8:21

> He will yet fill your mouth with laughter and your
> lips with shouts of joy.

REFLECTION

A negative attitude has a way of sneaking up on you from time to time. However, you are not supposed to remain in the hurt forever. Turn to Jesus when you are in a funk, He knows what it means to suffer. Jesus knows what it feels like to lose someone, what it is like to be hurt and how painful it is when someone betrays your trust. He endured many negativities during His time on earth and He does not want you to suffer like He did.

Instead, Jesus came so you could have life. He wants you to live your life to the fullest and enjoy all the best. He wants you to have abundance and journey through life with joy. This does not mean you ignore the negative feelings or put forth a false positive when you are suffering. It means to be grateful for all things, even the hard things. When you experience conflict or hurt, you need to allow yourself to feel them, but ask God to join you in the pain. It is in these moments when you can feel how powerful God is and how much He loves you.

Remember, God sent His only Son to earth so He could save the world (John 3:16). Jesus died so you might live and not just live but live abundantly (John 10:10). So, you need to do things which make you happy, make you laugh and that you enjoy. This is how you can give thanks to God for all He has given.

JOURNAL

Make a list of at least fifteen things that bring you joy and push yourself to grow the list to thirty things that make you happy. Push yourself to write down thirty things and try to do at least one every day, even if you do not feel like it. The purpose is to do one of these things every day to bring a little joy into your life. You deserve to have joy in your life every day.

Make a list of the things that bring you joy.

ACTION

As you stretch your body, also stretch your mind to think of more things that bring you joy.

Level 1: practice 15-20 minutes of yoga or stretching and do 15-20 minutes of a cross-training activity
Level 2: practice 20-40 minutes of yoga or stretching and do 20-40 minutes of a cross-training activity
Level 3: practice 30-60 minutes of yoga or stretching and do 30-60 minutes of a cross-training activity

Reflecting God

Scripture: 2 Corinthians 3:18

> And all of us, with unveiled faces, seeing the glory of the Lord as though reflected in a mirror, are being transformed into the same image from degree of glory to another for this comes from the Lord, the Spirit.

REFLECTION

It is common to be distracted by obligations. Full calendars can keep you busy from the time you get up until the time you lay down; then you start all over again. There is never time to look for God, but He is there even when you are not looking. God is there in each part of your day. He is everywhere you go, in the people and places. But today you will make time to slow down long enough to recognize God within yourself.

Stop to look at yourself in the mirror. Do not allow yourself to be drawn to the flaws, or what you perceive as flaws. Those are not flaws to God, but rather the things that make you unique in God's eyes. They may even be things those who love you think make you look like you. Let go of the negatives and allow yourself to be opened to see yourself as God sees you.

You are fearfully and wonderfully made in God's eyes (Ps 139:14). It is time you started to reflect the God that is within you. You might not always see Jesus in you or the beauty you are, but people do not love you because you are perfect, they love you because you are you. Today is the day when you are going to believe it.

JOURNAL

Look at yourself in the mirror and spend some time looking for God, looking for Jesus in your eyes. Do not allow yourself to only see the parts of you that you do not like, but instead look at yourself and see the creation God sees. He dwells in you; you are a tabernacle, and it is time you recognized the Jesus within you. After you look at yourself in the mirror for at least one minute, ultimately two minutes, write down what you see, think, and feel.

What do you see when you look into your eyes?

What thoughts do you have when you look yourself in your eyes?

How do you feel as you look into your own eyes?

Read what you wrote above and if there is anything negative, scratch out those words with a permanent marker. Do not let negative thoughts or feelings get stuck in your head. If you have negative thoughts and feelings about yourself, you are more likely to allow others to say them and believe them about yourself. God has great plans for you, and nothing is going to get in the way of what is in store, especially not things that are not true.

ACTION

Take time to do a little bit of light stretching before your exercise and remember to breathe deeply to connect with God through the breath.

> Level 1: walk 1-2 miles at a moderate pace
> Level 2: jog 2-4 miles at a moderate pace
> Level 3: run 3-7 miles at a moderate pace

DAY 54
Step Up
Scripture: Hebrews 11:1-3

> Now faith is the assurance of things hoped for, the conviction of things not seen. (Heb 11:1)

REFLECTION

So often you can get into a routine and become lazy. When you do the same thing over and over for a while, you just do not give it the same amount of effort as you did when you first began. Saint Paul is telling the Hebrews to build up their endurance and they will be successful Christians. This applies to you too, and this is what you are doing; both for the 5K and as a disciple. When you feel the routine beginning to get to be the same old stuff, change it up and step it up.

Disciples do not sit still they persevere whatever comes which builds endurance so they can be successful disciples. Jesus found the first disciples mending their nets, so they would be prepared to go out fishing the next day. It is an example to keep working, do not stand idle. Saint Paul warns of disciples becoming idle several times in scripture, including in 1 Timothy 5:13, 1 Thessalonians 5:14, and 2 Thessalonians 3:6, just to name a few.

If you have things that are challenging your faith right now, work it out. Find a way to find an answer or a way to sanctify it. Decide what you can do to live your faith more deeply. Identify how you can put your faith into action. You do not need to do something BIG but if you give your all to making a change, when combined with others doing the same thing, it can really make an impact.

JOURNAL

Disciples do not sit still, they act. Disciples are an example of love so you cannot just sit there and give love or show love. Love is a verb which means action. Set a goal today to run farther or faster than you have been. Make a note of what you have been doing so far both physically and spiritually.

Write down your physical actions.

Write down your spiritual actions.

ACTION

Reflect on the amount of effort you are putting forth during your exercise and your prayer time and decide if you are giving all you can or simply going through the motions to complete the task.

Level 1: spend 15-20 minutes doing yoga or stretching
and 20-30 minutes practicing a cross-training activity
Level 2: spend 20-40 minutes doing yoga or stretching
and 30-45 minutes practicing a cross-training activity
Level 3: spend 30-60 minutes doing yoga or stretching
and 45-60 minutes practicing a cross-training activity

On Purpose

Scripture: Genesis 2:2a

> And on the seventh day God finished the work that
> He had done.

REFLECTION

There are many people who take part in 5K races on a regular basis, and they have strategies or routines they follow to achieve their peak performance. They keep track of their regular runs and especially their races to strive towards their personal record, or PR. There are some who believe specific rituals leading up to the race gives them a boost or lays out the best possible conditions for them to hit a new PR. Since this is more than likely your first 5K, you do not have the experience that has taught you the best practices.

Some people will insist on going to bed at an early hour, some say to run or jog a one-mile course beforehand to warm up and, others will vow it is necessary to eat a big bowl of pasta the night before the race. Everyone you speak to will have a different suggestion about what you should do. There will be some who only walk, some who run and others who do a combination of the two. During the race you will meet people who will walk the hills and run the flat terrain. You will see people stop and visit with the volunteers who have the water station set up and others who will take the water and splash it in their face instead of drinking it.

If you choose to run a 5K race, you will encounter people who start the race off in a sprint and others who go at a steady pace. Then at the end of the race, you will find people who pick up the pace and sprint to the finish line, leaving you to wonder where that spurt of energy came from because they looked like they had already left everything on the course.

The practice of beginning to sprint when you see the finish line is not a disciple's philosophy. This practice of going harder at the end is not the mindset you need to make it to the cross. When your goal is to be a better disciple, you need to take it slowly so you can learn the lessons God wants you to learn and to spend time with those who need your time and attention. As you get closer to the goal, you might begin to get excited about reaching the goal and begin to work too hard. However, you want to remember to take time to rest, even God rested (Gen 2:3).

JOURNAL

On the seventh day, God rested. Rest is good. It is time to schedule something fun to do on your next rest day. When you are focused on a goal you can sometimes forget to have fun. Plan something great for your next day of rest and write down what you plan to do to relax. When you write things down you are more likely to remember them, so write it down and then do it.

> Write what you will do for fun on your next day of rest.

Also, as you begin to see the end of the challenge, start to think about what your next steps might be once you have completed *Discipleship 5K* and it is in your rearview mirror. You do not need to commit to anything right now, just consider the things you might continue to do, whether it is reading scripture or doing a specific type of exercise.

Write down your brainstorm ideas here so you have something to go back to later when it is time to decide.

ACTION

Stretch and breathe. These two simple things are often rushed through but if you do not complete the simple tasks, you will not be as practiced and disciplined. Be sure to do your stretching before and after your exercise. God is waiting to breathe with you.

Level 1: take a 2–4-mile leisurely walk
Level 2: take a 3–5-mile leisurely walk or jog
Level 3: take a 5–7-mile leisurely jog

DAY 56
Share Joy
Scripture: John 16:24

> Until now you have not asked for anything in my name. Ask and you will receive, so that your joy may be complete.

REFLECTION

Faith is not taught, it is caught. This is why disciples are called to go out and spread the good news. To share faith with others is called evangelization. Many people are not comfortable sharing their faith with others because they consider their faith to be too private and personal of a subject. However, it is in the job description of a disciple to share one's faith through words and action.

This does not mean you tell people how they should live their lives or how they should be going to church. This is not going to win friends or influence people. Your goal as a disciple is to spread the good news and be open to the good news from others. Allow others to share their faith with you and tell you where they see God in their lives. The Gospel message today is to ask God and He will make your joy complete. When you are full of God's grace and love you should be overflowing with joy and instead of simply letting your joy overflow, you must pass your joy on. Go out and share joy today!

JOURNAL

Tell someone who did not attend a church service this week about the message you heard. If the person you choose to speak to, did attend a church service, ask them about the sermon or homily at church or about the readings/scripture read and let them share their thoughts. Do not dominate the conversation, instead let them talk.

Write down what you learned through the scripture and what you heard them share. How will it apply to your life right now?

Write down what you learned.

Write down what the other person learned.

How will you apply what you learned to your life right now?

How does what the other person learned apply to your life right now?

ACTION

Keep up the great work! Your body is becoming stronger and more limber every day.

Level 1: practice 15-20 minutes of yoga or stretching and do 20-30 minutes of a cross-training activity
Level 2: practice 20-30 minutes of yoga or stretching and do 30-60 minutes of a cross-training activity
Level 3: practice 30-60 minutes of yoga or stretching and do 45-60 minutes of a cross-training activity

WEEK EIGHT OVERVIEW

Write down any thoughts, words of encouragement, ideas for growth or measurements of progress you have from this week from your physical and spiritual training.

WEEK NINE
Move Forward and Push Beyond

This week, the daily scripture will help to remind you that you began this challenge for a reason. You have a purpose, and you need to do whatever you can to stay motivated. Take time to figure out how you want to finish and what you will do to continue the work you have done. Remember, you are turning into a new creation.

As you begin week nine, it is like starting the third mile of your 5K. Today you can celebrate completing two-thirds of the challenge and that brings anticipation of seeing the finish line on the horizon. However, you still have another mile to go and this one might be the hardest yet. Even though by now the exercise and prayer time should be part of your routine, you will face obstacles. Do not get lazy. Stay vigilant. God has begun a good work in you, and He is there with you to see you to the end. You can do it!

Step by Step

Scripture: 2 Corinthians 9:11

> You will be enriched in every way for your great generosity, which will produce thanksgiving to God through us.

REFLECTION

You have something positive to contribute and today's scripture is a reminder of that fact. Over the past two months, you have been making sacrifices and doing the work. You have come so far both physically and spiritually. Today it is time to recognize how your behavior has changed and how it affects your attitude and how you treat others. You are doing hard things and have made progress; you need to celebrate.

A corner has been turned and as you begin the final month of training for the 5K there are some important things to remember.

1. You are not alone. In addition to your family and friends who are there each day, the *Discipleship 5K* community is here for you too. You are not the only person putting effort into building their physical and spiritual strength. Find the community on Facebook and Instagram for extra support and motivation; either by receiving it or giving it.

2. There are things you really like and there are things you do not like. At this point in the challenge, you know the things you look forward to doing and the things you procrastinate. Give yourself a break, and do not force yourself to do something you do not want to do. Now that you have the

habit of doing physical exercise, allow yourself to deviate a bit. As long as you are still moving your body and pushing yourself, the specific daily plan can be modified so you are spending your time doing the physical exercises that help you maintain a positive attitude.

3. You can do something, even if it is just a little bit and not as much as you think you need, you can still do something. This means on those days when something unexpected happens or interrupts your prayer time or exercise time, do not let it be a stressor. Instead, accept God's grace and find something positive that came from the distraction. For example, maybe a tree branch fell and knocked your mailbox down. You have no choice but to take care of removing the branch and resetting your mailbox. The time you spend getting this cleaned up will consume the time you had set aside to do your *Discipleship 5K* work. This could be devastating. Instead, set an alarm on your phone and every hour do ten jumping jacks or push-ups or sit-ups. It will not be equivalent to running or walking three miles or playing tennis or whatever your activity was for the day but at least you are doing something.

When you remember to do these things, it will affect your attitude in a positive way. The people around you will notice your behavior is different and it will cause others to want to do good things, too. It is all a part of learning how to see the world as God sees it. Look for the good, celebrate it and allow grace to fill the rest of the space. Let it be your little contribution to making the world a better place for everyone.

JOURNAL

It is week nine and you have accomplished so much. Write down 2-3 things you are proud of yourself for over the past couple of months. They can be things that pertain to *Discipleship 5K* or things that have happened at work or in a personal relationship. You have made some positive changes and it is a suitable time to reflect on all you have done. Keep giving your all, you are doing great!

Then going forward, at the end of each day, find something you can be proud of or happy about and do the 'happy dance.' Do you know that thing you do when you get good news or do something awesome? It is like your own little 'touchdown' celebration the NFL players do. Do you not have one? Get one! God is proud of you and you need to be proud of all you have done, too. It is time to do a 'happy dance' and celebrate you.

> Name 2-3 things you are proud of yourself for achieving.

ACTION

Remember to take time to stretch before and after your exercise.

> Level 1: walk 1-2 miles at a moderate pace
> Level 2: jog 2-4 miles at a moderate pace
> Level 3: run 3-7 miles at a moderate pace

DAY 58

Stay Encouraged

Scripture: 1 Thessalonians 3:6-13

> And may he so strengthen your hearts in holiness that you may be blameless before our God and Father at the coming of our Lord Jesus with all his saints. (1 Thess 3:13)

REFLECTION

Whether this is your first 5K training or your 101st, these final days of training begin to get mundane. You might have lost the zeal for the race; the excitement of the upcoming event has worn off and you have begun to let other things take priority over your training. Especially if you are doing this alone, you might feel like you are the only one who feels this way and you might even have thoughts of giving up. However, this scripture is meant to encourage you to keep on pushing because with each new day and new experience, you are growing in strength, hope and love.

As you begin the final month, you need to stay encouraged. There are times when you can see the end of the line and slow down because you see the end in sight. It is like when you are doing a plank and as you get to the end of your count to thirty, you start to count faster. At this point in the training, you do not have permission to give up. You need to hold strong. Stay motivated.

Take time to reflect on the past month, perhaps even look back to the end of the first month of the training. Then check in with yourself. What are things you do not look forward to? Remember you do not have to do them, but you need to find a comparable substitute so you can keep moving towards your goal. It is okay to change it up. The training to become a better disciple is not temporary, you are in it for the long haul so make sure it is fun. You are a living, breathing example of a disciple and through your words and actions, you are spreading the good news. If you are not feeling joyful about your training, you will not be reflecting joy and you will not have joy to share. Seek joy and it will begin to overflow in you.

JOURNAL

Look up some words of encouragement from saints and other famous people and make a list of thirty of them. Write down these words of wisdom, encouragement and inspiration in your journal and then make a copy of them. Cut them into strips so each piece of paper has one of the sayings on it. Then pick one from a jar or basket each day to read and allow the words to give you the encouragement to make it through the day. Let it be your daily mantra. You are amazing and these words will remind you of that fact.

What words of wisdom did you find and who said them? Write all of them here.

ACTION

Pick one of the strips of paper with the words of wisdom, encouragement, or inspiration to reflect on today as you stretch before your exercise.

> Level 1: participate in 10-15 minutes of a cross-training activity and spend 10-15 minutes doing a weight training activity
>
> Level 2: participate in 20-30 minutes of a cross-training activity and spend 10-15 minutes doing a weight training activity
>
> Level 3: participate in 60-90 minutes of a cross-training activity and spend 15-20 minutes doing a weight training activity

No Pain - No Gain

Scripture: Hebrew 12:11

> Now, discipline always seems painful rather than pleasant at the time, but later it yields the peaceful fruit of righteousness to those who have been trained by it.

REFLECTION

Jesus followed the laws of God, and His life was not without pain or challenges. There are many examples of Jesus's struggles throughout His public ministry beginning with the devil tempting Him in the desert (Matt 4:1-11) and ending with being crucified (Matt 27:32-44). Throw in the sadness He must have felt when Lazarus died (John 11:1-38) or when Judas betrayed Him (Matt 26:47-56), Jesus knows heartache.

Discipline is hard work and being a disciple requires discipline. The road to discipleship is plagued with disappointment, heartache, and loss. If Jesus had given the fishermen a job description of what it would take to follow Him, they probably would have remained there on the seashore. This is why looking to Jesus as a role model of someone who endured and persevered can help to keep you moving when the going gets tough.

Jesus knows there are good days and bad days, in life and in this challenge. He is there with you in both. When Jesus called your name to come and follow Him, He promised to be with you always (Matt 28:20), and that is something you can count on.

When you do have to deal with heartache or pain, Jesus will not judge you through the eyes of the world, rather through the eyes of

God. So, if you made some big strides in your physical training this week, but you slacked a bit on your spiritual training, Jesus is going to be happy with the effort you put forth and encourage you to do better next week. He is not in the business of making you feel guilty, instead Jesus is in the business of showing mercy and compassion.

You can read examples in the Bible of how Jesus did not always do everything the way He wanted to do it either, He was interrupted too. A few examples would be when He was on His way to see a little girl who had just died and was touched by a hemorrhaging woman (Matt 9:20-22) or when He and His disciples were getting in their boats to go pray, and the crowds came after them (Matt 14:13). Remember to give yourself some space for God's grace. Then you can begin anew each day, setting out to work harder and to do better.

The number one thing a disciple needs to do is to love God with all your heart, mind, and soul. The second thing is to learn discipline. This is the biggest lesson to learn through the physical and spiritual exercises of *Discipleship 5K*. Each day you are given tasks to conduct and along the way you learn how to trust, persevere, and do hard things. The scripture from Hebrews says discipline is painful, but over time you will see the good that comes from the arduous work. You are experiencing this firsthand.

In your life, you will have obstacles to overcome, and your true character is revealed through how you manage and overcome. This is what can be called the human experience. A good recipe to follow as you navigate through life is to maintain faith, stay positive and hold onto the hope that tomorrow will be better. All of it is a part of the transformation journey you are on to get to the cross.

JOURNAL

Take time to write a prayer to God asking specifically for the things you need to accomplish your goal. Then listen for God to respond. Remember prayer is a two-way conversation so allow space for God to give you hope, be a witness to the miracles of Christ and the strength to make things better.

Dear God,

AND/OR

Earlier in the challenge, you were asked to check in with a person who was also making a commitment to change a habit or learn a new behavior. It is time to ask how they are doing or how they did. Allow them to share their experience and then share your story. The purpose for checking in with them is not to boast about your positive changes or complain about the struggles; instead, this is an opportunity for you to connect with another person on a deeper level.

If you have stayed connected to this other person, then find a new person who has made the decision to make a change in their habits, whether joining the gym for the first time or beginning a new diet plan or deciding to spend more time in prayer. You might be surprised how easy it is to find someone who is trying to make a change in their life. Once you have found the person, do the same as above, ask them how they are doing and let them share their story before you jump in with your experience.

Write about the experience of checking in with your friend.

ACTION

Turn off the music, podcast or book you generally listen to while you stretch and allow that time of silence to be open for God to speak to you.

> Level 1: participate in 20-30 minutes of a cross-training activity
> Level 2: participate in 45-60 minutes of a cross-training activity
> Level 3: participate in 60-90 minutes of a cross-training activity

DAY 60

Turn Towards God

Scripture: Judges 2:10-15

> Moreover, that whole generation was gathered to their ancestors, and another generation grew up after them, who did not know the Lord or the world that he had done for Israel. (Judg 2:10)

REFLECTION

You are not the only one struggling with putting God first. Everyone struggles with the temptations of the world. It is a problem as old as Adam and Eve. The scripture today is one example. God does not want you to feel pressured into being a disciple. He gives you the choice to follow him. Of course, He wants you to turn towards Him, but He will not force you.

It is hard to keep up the discipline needed to be a good disciple all the time. Taking the easy road can be very tempting at times. Especially when doing the right thing could cause divisions in relationships, primarily with those who have authority over you or of your time. It can be equally frustrating when someone tells you what they think is best for you to do or tries to make you do something you know is wrong. It can feel as though they are making you do it because they have created consequences you will face if you do not do what they demand you do.

The people in the Old Testament did not always follow God's Law. They liked to do things their own way and then when they got into trouble, they would blame God for not rescuing them from the pain or suffering the consequences of their own decisions. It is a situation most everyone experiences at one time or another.

Instead of turning away from God because you are hurting or do not understand, try to turn towards God. The Bible is full of stories about how God helps people find a way through even the most terrifying situations.

When you look at your progress and participation in *Discipleship 5K,* there might be things you are frustrated about, and you might even get mad at yourself or God. You might think the progress you have made getting to your goals is due to the sacrifices you have made and that would be true, but you have to remember God is there too. When you look back on the amount of time you have dedicated, the things you have sacrificed, you can look back in your journal and see how much you have changed physically and spiritually. A disciple will see God's hand in it the entire time. You do not always see God in the picture but let this scripture be a reminder to you that He is there even if you turn your back.

God asks for your obedience. He does not force it. Today, is a wakeup call to get on track for this final leg of the race.

JOURNAL

Today, follow God's example and pray for people with whom you do not agree or have different beliefs or opinions. God might be able to help shine light on the situation. The best way to find perspective is through prayer. Pray to God for understanding and pray for understanding for a person or person with whom you have a conflict or difference of opinion. Allow God to help you both come to a solution you can agree upon.

Spend at least 10-15 minutes in prayer, focused specifically on someone who is in a position of authority with whom you have trouble following. Pray for insight on why you have a conflict and for that person to gain understanding as well. Write down your thoughts and insight. Allow God to open you up to understand and to be understood.

Write a summary of your prayer.

ACTION

Practice breathing for 5-10 minutes. As you breathe, think about the person you are having a conflict with and identify at least five positive attributes about that person.

> Level 1: spend 15-20 minutes doing yoga or stretching and 20-30 minutes of a cross-training activity
> Level 2: spend 20-40 minutes doing yoga or stretching and 30-45 minutes of a cross-training activity
> Level 3: spend 30-60 minutes doing yoga or stretching and 45-60 minutes of a cross-training activity

Push Yourself

Scripture: Proverbs 2:8

> Guarding the paths of justice and preserving the
> way of his faithful ones.

REFLECTION

The scripture today says to guard the paths of justice and preserve
the way of the faithful. That is a tough thing to do sometimes. Take
a minute to think about the examples in your life, of people who
stand up for you or for what is right, every time. Is it a parent? A
sibling? A best friend? Today you want to look for the people, who
for the most part, do the right thing and then figure out what you
can learn from their example.

When you think of the people who you know are in your corner,
the ones who take care of you, and help ensure you are protected, pay
attention to how they make you feel. Generally, that bigger than life
feeling is something people try to hide for fear of being thought of as
egotistic or boastful. Instead, use this feeling to inspire you to push
yourself harder, to go further and to run faster. Sometimes you can
believe you are giving it all you have, but then you imagine working
harder for someone who means a lot to you and miraculously you
have the strength to give a little more. In these moments you can
find yourself pulling energy from someplace you cannot reach on
your own.

Perhaps there is someone who you have never met who inspires
you to be a better person. Maybe you heard about their story on the
news or in a book and their ability to push through inspired you.
There are several movies, based on or inspired by actual events that

can make everyone in the theatre want to give more and be better. Find yours.

God has placed in you a level of strength that you cannot get to on your own. There are times when you can only push your limits for someone else. Like in the stories where you hear of mothers who have the strength to lift a car off their child so they can escape being trapped inside. In these instances, the mothers would tell you that they just did what they had to do for their children or someone they love. First Responders push themselves for total strangers every day.

God pushed Himself by giving His only Son as a sacrifice. Then Jesus lived out the sacrifice. Jesus was able to push Himself through all the pain and suffering so He could get to the cross. Jesus was pushing Himself harder because of you. As a disciple you need to push yourself too. You need to find those people who you are willing to work harder for and make for sacrifices in your life. They might even be people you have never met.

JOURNAL

Try to go a little harder to see what you can achieve today. While you do this, think of those who are examples for you, people who go the extra mile to help or support you and others. Everyone needs those examples to help stay motivated and trust that the world is really a nice place. Allow them to be an inspiration to you as you go through the rest of this challenge. Who will you lean on to push you when you need a boost?

> Write down 2-3 people in your life whose strength
> and perseverance inspire you. Identify the specific
> obstacle they overcame or the strength they showed

to persevere and use their story to push you as you continue the journey to the cross.

Identify 2-3 movies that have given you that, 'anything is possible' feeling. Refer to these stories when you need an extra boost to make it to your goal.

ACTION

Remember to spend time before and after your exercise doing your breathing and stretching. Also, push yourself to do a little extra and add 10 minutes of calisthenics to your routine.

Level 1: walk 1.5-2 miles as fast as you can
Level 2: run 2-3.5 miles at your peak pace
Level 3: run 4-8 miles at your peak pace

Remain Faithful

Scripture: 2 Kings 2:11

> As they continued walking and talking, a chariot
> of fire and horses of fire separated the two of them,
> and Elijah ascended in a whirlwind into heaven.

REFLECTION

Being a disciple when things are going well is easy but when dreadful
things happen, it can be a struggle. God puts people in your path
to help you through tough times. He provides you with a support
group from the moment you are born; it is called a family.

Additionally, there are people in your life God puts in your path for
a specific reason. Some are there to walk with, to learn from and to lean
on for only a season of your life and others are there throughout your
lifetime. Each of these people have been put in your path for a different
reason. There could be people you know very well, while others you
simply know their names, but when you walk together and listen to
one another, you are being Christ to one another. You never know what
God has planned or who you might learn something from in life. You
could gain great wisdom from someone you meet one time and other
times a person who once was a stranger, become a mentor or guide.

Today's scripture shares a specific moment in time when Elijah
and Elisha, prophets from the Old Testament experience a defining
moment. Elijah, who had been called to mentor Elisha is taken
to heaven and Elisha is left there alone. After years of traveling
together, where Elijah taught Elisha the ropes, they are a wonderful
example of apprenticeship. Then, without warning, God reunites
Elijah with Himself, and Elisha is left to pick up and continue the

work. Thankfully, Elijah and Elisha were like family, and they had built a faith community who loved them and supported them in good times and in bad.

When Elijah was taken to heaven, Elisha could have stopped the work they had been doing. He could have used it as an excuse to quit. Not only is this scripture a story of two men who supported one another like family through thick and thin, but also a story of how even in pain and suffering, you must continue to persevere. Do not let this training just stop when you finish the book. Like Elisha, you will still have work to do even when the 5K has been completed.

JOURNAL

Reflect today on the people who have made a lasting impact on your life, influenced you, or encouraged you to be a better human being. They are the key to you staying faithful to the challenge and beyond. Also note, you can list more than one person if you have had more than one mentor in your lifetime; they do not need to be actively mentoring you right now.

Who do you consider a mentor?

Inspired by the scripture to walk the path of life with someone, reach out to another person you know who is training or has made a commitment to change their routine and see if you can train together today or this week.

To whom will you reach out?

ACTION

Today's journal requires some real reflection. While you stretch, reflect on the people who have served as a mentor to you in your life. If the person is alive and lives near you, perhaps they can join you on your walk today. If not, reflect on the things you might have discussed while on your walk.

Level 1: take a 2–4-mile leisurely walk
Level 2: take a 3–5-mile leisurely walk or jog
Level 3: take a 5–7-mile leisurely jog

Prepare

Scripture: Matthew 24:44

> Therefore, you also must be ready, for the Son of
> Man is coming at an unexpected hour.

REFLECTION

There is no promise of tomorrow. God can come at any time. Are you ready? You have been preparing for over two months and it is time to get yourself in the mindset to be ready. Think of Elisha from yesterday's scripture, and how he was prepared to continue pushing forward towards the goal he and Elijah had even though Elisha was going to have do it on his own. Elisha did what he needed to, even though it was difficult.

So, are you ready? What if the 5K race was tomorrow, how prepared would you be? It is time to decide if you are ready to complete the race in the same way you were when you began this training. Perhaps you need to make some adjustments to your expectations. Maybe you need to schedule a couple of extra trainings over the next few weeks. You do not want race day to sneak up on you and you not be prepared to accomplish your goal.

JOURNAL

Take time to consider what you need to do to be more motivated. How can you change up your routine to keep you focused on the training? Not only do you need to stay focused and motivated on your physical training but also your spiritual training. You want to be ready when Jesus comes.

> What two things will you do to stay motivated physically?

> What two things will you do to stay motivated spiritually?

It is also time to prepare for what is going to happen once you complete the race and this book. Start to brainstorm what kind of things you might do to stay connected spiritually once the discipleship training is completed. Research bible studies or other classes or groups you could take part in to stay motivated in practicing your faith at a deeper level. Write down your ideas.

ACTION

Imagine the various ways you can incorporate prayer more deeply into your exercise time. Do your yoga or stretching in silence to allow God to contribute to the list.

> Level 1: do 15-20 minutes of yoga or stretching and take part in 30-45 minutes of a cross-training activity
> Level 2: do 20-30 minutes of yoga or stretching and take part in 45-60 minutes of a cross-training activity
> Level 3: do 30-60 minutes of yoga or stretching and take part in 60-90 minutes of a cross-training activity

WEEK NINE OVERVIEW

Write down any thoughts, words of encouragement, ideas for growth or measurements of progress you have from this week from your physical and spiritual training.

WEEK TEN
Connect with Yourself

Over the past nine weeks you have worked hard to build a deeper relationship with God. You have also reached out to peers checking in on them and praying for them. At times it may have been a tough road, but it all has been worth the effort. Instead of focusing on your relationship with God or with others, this week, take care of yourself. Now is not the time to give up or push too hard and suffer an injury or be distracted from the goal at hand. Take time to recharge, refresh, and reach inside yourself to find out what you need to make it through the next few weeks and finish strong.

It might feel strange for you to pamper yourself with a foot soak or to schedule a massage. This notion to pause to check in with yourself might seem like the opposite of what you should do with only three weeks until the race. Maybe you are beginning to feel anxious or overwhelmed just thinking about taking time for yourself when there is so much to do. Do not allow yourself to be worried about what is going to happen in the future. Instead, focus on the present.

Remember, God's ways are not the ways of the world. And so, when the world says, you cannot take a break, God says you need to give yourself some grace. Race day is around the corner which makes it the perfect time for you to take a breath, check in with yourself and how you are doing physically and spiritually right now, in the present. Think of it as a thank you gift for all your dedication and sacrifice over the past nine weeks.

Make plans to do something you have not allowed yourself the time to do since you began this challenge. Some suggestions might be to designate 30 minutes to lay on the couch and read a book, or you need to schedule a date night or happy hour with your friends. It may even be something as simple as putting on a mud mask and trimming your toenails. You deserve to take time for yourself. It is time to practice self-love.

DAY 64

Random Acts of Kindness

Scripture: Psalm 14:1-7

> The Lord looks down from heaven on humankind
> to see if there is any who are wise, who seek after
> God. (Ps 14:2)

REFLECTION

The scripture today is the entire chapter of Psalm 14. It explains that the people are losing sight of God, and no one is doing anything good for God or for one another. This happens in the world today as well. It happens all the time. You can go several days in a row without seeing any display of Christian love in the world. Unfortunately, you have probably fallen victim to it too because it is easy to get consumed with expectations and obligations of the world and not give glory or honor to God.

So, as you give yourself time to refresh and rejuvenate by doing something fun or special this week, remember that you cannot give what you do not have. This means you must be feeding yourself, filling your fuel tank so that when you are called on to help a neighbor, you are ready to help them because you have something to give. The scripture says the people lost sight of God's plan for them which means you must do the opposite; you need to find ways to connect and keep the connection to God.

There is an old song that says, 'they will know you are Christian by your love.' When you are Christ to one another, then you are following Jesus' example to treat others as you would like to be treated. Go out and be an example of Christ in the world so people do not lose hope that God is here. Mother Teresa said, "God has no feet but your feet and no hands but your hands." And further, Saint Francis of Assisi said to "speak the Gospel at all times and if necessary, use words." Both phrases express a beautiful invitation to show others the love and charity of Christ through words and actions.

Fill yourself up with Christ. Look for His presence everywhere you go. Then if you cannot find Him, be Christ for others. It is like a smile and it contagious.

JOURNAL

Do a random act of kindness or pay it forward and watch how God is revealed in your actions. It can be as simple as holding the door open for someone or making eye contact with a stranger as you say 'Hello.' Perhaps go a bit deeper and ask someone how their day is going and pause to genuinely listen to their response. Sometimes you will hear of a random act of kindness that happened in a drive thru line where a customer pays for the order of the car behind them. Kindness is kindness.

What random act of kindness will you share today to fill yourself up?

ACTION

Ask a friend to join you in your cross-training activity today. If the class has a fee, pay for them. If it does not have a fee, offer to take them for coffee or a smoothie afterwards, your treat.

Level 1: give your all doing 20-30 minutes of a cross-training activity
Level 2: give your all doing 45-60 minutes of a cross-training activity
Level 3: give your all doing 60-90 minutes of a cross-training activity

New Hope

Scripture: Ezekiel 36:24-28

> A new heart I will give you, a new spirit I will put within you; and I will remove from your body the heart of stone and give you a heart of flesh. (Ezek 36:26)

REFLECTION

The purpose of the 5K and discipleship training is to build you up; give you strength in faith to persevere and accomplish much. The hope and desire at the end of the twelve weeks is that you will have become a new creation in Christ. The desire is that you become someone who has a deeper relationship with Jesus.

In the passage from Ezekiel, God is taking you and leading you to the place He wants you to go. He gives you a clean heart, a fresh start so you can begin again. Imagine someone who's heart is failing and gets weaker every day, then someone comes along to give them a new heart. What joy they would feel!

This is what God is doing for you as well. It is a lot of work but each day you face new challenges physically and spiritually and you are getting stronger. God gives you something to look forward to, a new motivation to push you to the next level. This is great news.

JOURNAL

Allow God to give you new motivation, new hope as you reflect on the ways you have changed over the past several weeks.

How has God given you a new heart or made you into a new creation?

Reflect on how you have been cleansed through this training. Do you see and/or feel differences within yourself? What has changed and do you like this change? Why or why not?

ACTION

Remember to schedule time to stretch and practice your breathing techniques before and after your exercises today.

Level 1: participate in 10-15 minutes of a cross-training activity and 10-15 minutes of a weight training activity

Level 2: participate in 20-30 minutes of a cross-training activity and 10-15 minutes of a weight training activity

Level 3: participate in 60-90 minutes of a cross-training activity and 15-20 minutes of a weight

Self-Care

Scripture: Exodus 15:26

> He said, 'If you will listen carefully to the voice of the Lord your God, and do what is right in his sight, and give heed to his commandments and keep all his statutes, I will not bring upon you any of the diseases that I brought upon the Egyptians; for I am the Lord who heals you.'

REFLECTION

God reminds the Israelites to follow the Ten Commandments and He will not send the plagues or locusts or any of the other things He put on Pharaoh. It is a bit of a threat but sometimes these little reminders are needed to stay on track. God wants you to keep His Commandments and when you do so, He will support you. This is the promise He made to the Israelites, and He promises you this too.

The Commandments say to love God, and through your participation in *Discipleship 5K* you are showing your love for God by spending time in prayer and reflecting on His presence in your life. They also say to love others, and you are doing this by praying for others and taking part in random acts of kindness. You are also expressing gratitude to those who support you and letting them know you appreciate their positive influence. These activities have given you opportunities to follow the Commandments.

However, you cannot forget to show love for yourself too. It is easy to get wrapped up with meeting the needs of others and praying for them, then forget to care for your own needs. Sometimes it can feel embarrassing to admit that you need prayer and healing because it can feel like a sign of weakness. But remember, Jesus said to love your neighbor as yourself, so you must also be taking care of satisfying your needs. If you do not take the time to care for yourself, you might not have the energy to care for others when they reach out for help. Therefore, it is time to take care of yourself this week; you might be putting on a good show, allowing others to believe you are doing great, when in fact you are hurting. Surrender.

If you let a little blister, go, it will turn into a big blister and could pop. It is time to take care of any maintenance things you may have been putting off such as trimming your toenails or getting a haircut. Maybe you have been putting off mowing your lawn or calling your mom. Perhaps the thing that will fill you the most right now is going to watch your granddaughter's dance class, which was something you used to do regularly before you began the activities in *Discipleship 5K*. Whatever it is, God will provide you with the time to do the things you need to do because you are doing the things, He wants you to do.

JOURNAL

God says if you follow his commandments, He will take care of you in return. Today, the journal exercise reflects God's example of 'if you take care of me, then I'll take care of you.' Write out your prayers as petitions to God, which identifies who and what you wish God to give special attention to today. Begin with the people in your life who need physical or spiritual healing. If you do not have specific people in your life who need this type of prayer, you can pray for groups of people who are in need, such as refugees or homeless or people battling cancer, etc. Turn on the news if you do not know anyone who needs prayer, and you will find several people who could use someone to pray for them. Remember, Saint Paul told the Philippians to pray in this way too, making their petitions known to God (Phil 4:6) because it is good pray for the needs for others and not only for yourself.

Write your petitions to God.

If you can, take your prayer a step further by putting it into action. Do one special thing for each person you wrote a petition for in the previous exercise. Write down what you will do.

ACTION

Spend 5-10 minutes stretching before and after your exercise. Also do 10-20 minutes of calisthenics to work on muscle groups that do not get exercise when you walk or run.

Level 1: walk 1.5-2 miles as fast as you can
Level 2: run 2-3.5 miles at your peak pace
Level 3: run 4-8 miles at your peak pace

DAY 67
Self-Love

Scripture: 2 Timothy 2:22-26

> Pursue righteousness, faith, love, and peace. (2 Tim 2:22)

REFLECTION

There may be times when you get down on yourself and lose sight of the good things you do or do not give yourself credit when credit is due. It is so much easier to pick out the bad than to focus on the good. If the journal activity invited you to make a list of ten things that you have NOT done well today, you would probably be able to make the list quickly without much thought. The negative is easier to believe and to remember. However, when you spend too much time focused on the things you have done wrong, you become vulnerable to the tricks of the devil.

Instead, practice looking at yourself as God sees you. It might feel a little strange because when you look at yourself as God looks at you, there is an amazing person who has many wonderful gifts to share staring at you in the mirror. This can be awkward because the world says that you should not go around boasting about your accomplishments.

In the world today, if you say you are good at something and draw attention to it, you are perceived as boastful and overconfident. However, the world does not define who you are, God does. And God wants you to use the gifts you have been given to show His glory. You are called to share the things you do well with others and to teach them about God's goodness. You must learn how to give yourself permission to share your gifts and to love yourself. God calls you to love your neighbor as yourself and if you do not have love of self, loving others can be difficult.

Remember God's ways are not the ways of the world. So, when the world says you are selfish, overconfident, and self-righteous because you love yourself, then let them say it. Taking care of yourself and working on yourself does not make you selfish, it makes you self-aware. When you love yourself, the love you have for others will grow because it will have depth and meaning that can only come from letting the Spirit of God dwell in you. Then you can see each thing God created as good, including yourself.

JOURNAL

First write a definition of self-love. Then name 5-10 things that you love about yourself and really aim to come up with ten things. If you need help, ask God to tell you what He loves about you and allow God to help make your list by looking at yourself as God sees you. It may be difficult, but it is necessary for you to learn how to give yourself love and acknowledge your goodness without feeling selfish. You should be proud of your accomplishments and celebrate the things that make you the unique creation God intends you to be.

Write the definition of self-love in your own words.

Make a list of 10 things you love about yourself.

ACTION

Practice breathing for 5-10 minutes. As you breathe, think about the things other people have said that they love about you and compare what they said to what you wrote down during your journal time.

> Level 1: practice 15-20 minutes of yoga or stretching and take part in 20-30 minutes of a cross-training activity
> Level 2: practice 20-40 minutes of yoga or stretching and take part in 30-45 minutes of a cross-training activity
> Level 3: practice 30-60 minutes of yoga or stretching and take part 45-60 minutes of a cross-training activity

Sacrifice

Scripture: Hebrews 10:1-18

> When he said above, "You have neither desired nor
> taken pleasure in sacrifices and offerings and burnt
> offerings and sin offerings." (Heb 10:8)

REFLECTION

Maybe when you hear the word sacrifice you think of something terrible. The word sacrifice can carry a negative connotation when you think of someone dying for the sake of another person. But sacrifice is not a bad word.

In baseball, a player is sometimes called upon to sacrifice bunt. This is a strategy for the team to gain a better position to score a run. The goal is for the batter to sacrifice his at bat so he can advance the runner(s) for the good of the team. In this case, the sacrifice is a good thing because it helps the entire team. The player sacrifices his at bat for the greater good. Jesus did this too.

Sacrificing something for the greater good is not so bad; many say it is even worth it. Jesus sacrificed himself as one final sacrifice for the good of all people. He gave his life so sins would be forgiven. Jesus' sacrifice is honored, celebrated, and remembered. He died so you and I could be saved from sin and have eternal life. One sacrifice to save us all. What a game changer!

JOURNAL

You have made sacrifices so you could take part in *Discipleship 5K*. Take time to reflect and consider how the time and energy you have sacrificed has been for good. Identify what good has come through your sacrifice physically and spiritually.

> How has your time and energy been sacrificed physically?

> How has your time and energy been sacrificed spiritually?

> Would you agree the sacrifices you have made have been good? Explain.

> How would your family and/or friends respond to this question?

ACTION

Remember to take time to stretch and practice your breathing.

> Level 1: walk 1-2 miles at a moderate pace
> Level 2: jog 2-4 miles at a moderate pace
> Level 3: run 3-7 miles at a moderate pace

Keep Moving

Scripture: 2 Thessalonians 3:6-13

> Keep away from believers who are living in idleness
> and not according to the tradition. (2Thess 3:6b)

REFLECTION

Idleness is a sin, and the scripture is a reminder of this fact. Saint Paul is warning the Thessalonians against standing still as well as from spending time with people who are not putting in the work of living out the faith they proclaim. This warning is for you too. You want to be ready, willing, and able to do what God calls you to do as a disciple, there is no time to just sit around. This is not saying that you cannot take a break or do something good for yourself. It is saying, do not sit still and expect the same results as when you are putting in the work.

This is equally important physically and spiritually. There are physically noticeable differences when you get lackadaisical about your workout routine such as, your pants do not button up as easily and your shirt fits around your chest or tummy a bit too tightly. These are things you can see.

When you get lazy in your prayer life, there are not the visual reminders. Instead, imagine that each time you put something before your time with God, you are putting a block in between you and God. Sometimes you can still see God and feel close to Him, but after you put three or five or ten things before God, it becomes much more difficult to see or feel the closeness you did when you spent time with Him daily.

This challenge has taught you so much about motivation and working hard; this is when you need to be putting it into practice.

You need to navigate the roadblocks, anticipate the obstacles, and think through possible action steps so you are prepared to overcome anything that might get in your way. Remember to reach out for motivation and encouragement from all sides. Idleness is a sin which means you have to keep moving.

Set yourself up for success and do not let little distractions keep you from achieving your goal. You have come too far to get distracted by others who do not understand the commitment you have made. It is important to keep a good balance of work and leisure but do not be tempted to get lazy in these last weeks of preparation. Remember you are becoming a new creation, there are new norms your friends, family and coworkers are going to have to get used to when they spend time with you. Do not conform; be transformed (Rom 12:2).

JOURNAL

This choice to be a disciple is not really a choice. It is something God calls all His creation to become, and you have chosen to do it in a deliberate, intentional way through *Discipleship 5K*. So, as you go about your day, think about how you can be an example to others and motivate them to actively choose to follow Jesus and be a disciple too.

Where is God calling you to be of service to others?

Make a list of at least three things you can do to serve in your community.

Write down at least five specific actions you can take to inspire others. Consider how you can do this in your personal life with your family, at work or in your community.

ACTION

Allow yourself at least 30 minutes of silence as you walk or jog so you can listen to God's direction for where He wants you to serve.

Level 1: take a 2–4-mile leisurely walk and spend 10-15 minutes doing yoga or stretching
Level 2: take a 3–5-mile leisurely walk or jog spend and 15-20 minutes doing yoga or stretching
Level 3: take a 5–7-mile leisurely jog and spend 20-30 minutes doing yoga or stretching

Ask - Seek - Knock

Scripture: Matthew 7:7

> Ask, and it will be given you; search, and you will
> find; knock, and the door will be opened for you.

REFLECTION

Today's scripture comes from the Gospel of Matthew, chapter 7, verse 7. Symbolically, the number 7 is an especially important number in scripture, as are the numbers 3 and 12. So, today, as you read the Word of God, be extra mindful of the words of the scripture and what message God is sending to you right now. There might be something extra special for you to hear.

Plus, this passage is a popular one, so chances are you have heard these words before or even have it memorized and quote it. However, these words of scripture, though very simple and specific, can be hard to believe and a challenge to live out.

Ask. Search. Knock. God says all you need to do is ask and it will be given to you. This sounds easy enough to do, but God wants you to ask for what you want and what you feel/believe/think you need, but what you ask for is not always what God believes is best for you at that time. This first step of asking God can cause some trouble in your thinking because you have been taught and scripture confirms that God already knows what you need. It can sound contradictory to have to ask God. Do not get tripped up on this. When you think God already knows what you need, it can keep you from going through the formality of asking; naming what it is you want/need God to provide for you in this moment. It can keep you from praying because if God knows already, then what is the point in asking? Further, if you ask for something and it is not God's will for it or it is not the right time, then it can get frustrating to ask for anything for fear you will never get it.

Today society is all about instant gratification with fast food and instant messaging. Modern technology does not leave room for patience, everything comes quickly, often instantly. It can be very frustrating when God does not respond to your request right away. The scripture clearly says, all you must do is ask and the door will be opened. However, God does not always open the door in the way you expect Him to. Sometimes God's answer does come instantly but you chose to ignore it or since it is not the answer you expect, you keep your mind closed to the possibility of it working the way God proposes.

So, even if you do ask, the second step of searching and finding the answer can get confusing. You can get trapped in the 'what you think is best vs. what God thinks is best merry-go-round.' Unfortunately, this ride is one every human being in the history of the world has taken a trip on a time or two. You might even think God is paying hide and seek, but God is not playing games, even though it can feel that way when He does not show up in the way you expect or within your timeframe.

Once you reach the decisive step and you find yourself standing in front of the door where the answer is on the other side, you can become paralyzed. There are times when what you ask for, you are not ready to accept. You might stand there outside the door for a long time before you are called to reach out and open it. It is one of the hardest parts of faith, trusting in God's timing.

JOURNAL

The message is asked, and you will receive, knock and the door will be opened. It is a popular verse, but human experience says this is not true. This is the reason it is such an important verse. God needs you to communicate with Him and trust that He knows what is best for you.

How often do you find yourself waiting on God's timing?

How well do you wait for God's response when you ask for something?

It requires faith and trust that God will give you what you need when you need it. Ask God to help lighten the stress and burden you carry in your life. Ask with a grateful heart and then wait for God to respond. Write out your prayer to God, ask for what you need.

Dear God,

ACTION

As you practice your breathing and you do your stretches, think of the things you have waited on this week and thank God for the opportunities to practice your patience.

> Level 1: practice 15-20 minutes of yoga or stretching and take part in 30-45 minutes of a cross-training activity

Level 2: practice 20-30 minutes of yoga or stretching and take part in 45-60 minutes of a cross-training activity

Level 3: practice 30-60 minutes of yoga or stretching and take part in 60-90 minutes of a cross-training activity

WEEK TEN OVERVIEW

Write down any thoughts, words of encouragement, ideas for growth or measurements of progress you have from this week from your physical and spiritual training.

WEEK ELEVEN
M&M – Maintenance and Mindset

The end goal is near, and it is time to check in with yourself. The two things to focus on this week are the M&M's! No, not the melt in your mouth, not in your hand candy. Although, the M&M candy might be just what you need to finish these final two weeks strong. Today you get to decide exactly what you will need to make it to the finish line. This week you will check on the two M's, Maintenance and Mindset.

Maintenance is a word that means 'upkeep.' When you own a car or home, there is regular maintenance you must do to keep them doing what you need them to do. For a car it means putting good gas in the tank and changing the oil regularly. For a home it looks like changing the air filter, the batteries in your smoke detectors and checking the gutters to make sure all the gunk is cleaned out of them. These are things you must do to keep the car and home in decent shape. For you and your body, it means making sure you are eating well, getting good sleep and that all your body parts are showing up in good health so they can do their job of keeping you in the race; both figuratively and literally.

Maintenance also means 'the support of' so you need to check in with the things you need to support you over the next few weeks. Perhaps you have a favorite pair of running shoes, but they are wearing thin. You need to be realistic whether those shoes will help you be your best self on race day. Maybe they need to take a break and you need to train in the second-string pair of shoes so your favorite pair can take a little time off. You need to figure out what helps you perform the best and you need to make those factors happen. There are some people who like to carry water and others that do not like the extra weight, some like to wear a hat and others who say that it makes them hot and sweat more. These things can be distractions and could cause frustration which is what you should try to avoid. This week, your goal is to find the conditions that provide you with the best-case scenario for success.

And Mindset. This is equally important because you need to make sure your mind is on the right track. You need to have a clear goal. You need to be focused and have everything ready so you can be the most effective as you can. This means setting yourself up for success now instead of waiting until the day of the race or for the last day of the challenge.

You need to imagine yourself getting up on the morning of the race and imagining step-by-step what you will need. Know what you are going to wear, know what you will eat, decide what your prerace routine will be. These are the things that can trip you up and cause you to go off course if you do not think them through. If you signed up for an actual 5K or other race, you might want to go back and check the registration to see when and where you pick up your race packet and maybe even review the race path. Taking time to review the race path ahead of race day can help you study the terrain. Looking ahead gives you the opportunity to find the hills that might slow you down and allow time to wrap your mind around some of the things that could trip you up. When you prepare ahead of time, then your mind will already be trained, and you will be less likely to tell yourself to simply quit because it is too hard. Instead, you will already be aware of some of the obstacles that lay ahead, and you will be ready to overcome them when you come face to face.

Another thing that could be helpful in making sure your mind is ready is to spend 5-10 minutes in meditation each day imagining yourself filling a bucket with all the stressful things going on in your life so on race day, you can put the bucket aside as you work to complete your goal. Throughout the challenge, you have been taking strides to change your mindset, to think more like a disciple. You have been training to be strong and persevere. You want to do whatever you can to stay positive and see yourself finishing strong. As you near the end of the challenge, you are going to put these things to the test and this week the exercises will help ensure you will be ready.

DAY 71

Stand Tall

Scripture: 2 Timothy 1:6-13

> For this reason I remind you to rekindle the gift of God that is within you through the laying on of my hands; for God did not give us a spirit of cowardice, but rather a spirit of power and of love and of self-discipline. (2Tim 1:6-7)

REFLECTION

Be sure to take out your Bible and read the entire scripture passage. There are some particularly important words Saint Paul is sharing with Timothy. Remember, Timothy is a young leader in the community of new Christians, so Paul is often reminding him of his worthiness. In this piece of scripture, Paul tells Timothy that God did not give him the spirit of cowardice, rather the spirit of power and self-discipline. He goes on to tell him to rely on the power of God because he has been called to fulfill a purpose and it is through that power the purpose is revealed. Then Paul tells Timothy to guard the treasure that has been entrusted to him.

These words from Saint Paul are not unique to Timothy. They are written as a reminder and a promise for each and every child of God. They clearly state the purpose for which you have been called and God will be there with you to complete the task. What an important and relevant piece of scripture as you begin the final two weeks of *Discipleship 5k*!

Stand tall and be proud of the accomplishments thus far, you have done a lot. Even if you have hit a few bumps along the way, you are still here and doing the work. You have worked extremely hard to get this far on the journey. Do not let anyone tell you that it has not been worth it, nor should you feel embarrassed about your participation in the training. You need to be proud to be a follower of Jesus. Do not be ashamed. When you show up and give your best, God knows it and He will get you the rest of the way to fulfilling your purpose.

It is the same for being a disciple. Remember, Peter denied Jesus three times, and yet he became the first Pope of the Catholic Church. God has a plan for you and even though you might take some detours and even though there are highs and lows, difficulties to endure, God is there. This scripture, and honestly the entire Bible is a good reminder to keep a spirit of power, love, and self-discipline, especially when you do not feel you have enough energy to finish. Look at the examples of those who struggled in the Bible and overcame great odds. It is your turn to stand tall and be proud of all you have accomplished. Even on the days when you can only give 40%, God will show up with the remaining 60%.

JOURNAL

Read the scripture passage, then write a sentence or two naming how God's Word makes you feel. Then call, text, or tell someone in person about the passage and how it speaks to you right now.

How does the scripture make you feel?

Who are you going to call, text or tell in person about this scripture passage?

ACTION

Practice your deep breathing and spend time before and after your exercise stretching to help prevent injury.

> Level 1: walk 1.5-3 miles at a moderate pace
> Level 2: jog 2-4 miles at a moderate pace
> Level 3: run 4-8 miles at a moderate pace

DAY 72

Good Work

Scripture: Philippians 2:13

> For it is God who is at work in you, enabling you both to will and to work for his good pleasure.

REFLECTION

The scripture today is so beautiful. It says God is giving you the will and the work to fulfill your purpose. Wow! It is so refreshing to hear, God created you for a purpose and He will see you through to completion. This is great news, right?

But you still need to stay motivated to have the will and you need to know the endgame so you can work towards it. It can be hard to stay motivated if you do not know what the goal is, especially if it is not specific. This is one of the reasons *Discipleship 5K* was created, because there are times in life when the endgame is clear like, to complete a 5K and other times when it is simply to survive another day. In either case, you cannot do it alone on your own will, rather you need God's Will to complete the task in front of you so you can live your best life as a disciple, a child of God.

Whatever God wills for you, will be seen to completion. These words of scripture give strength and hope on those debilitating days when you are not hitting the mark. The scripture today, like yesterday is supposed to be a motivator. Remember God sees differently than you see, so when you see failure and laziness, God fills you with grace and mercy, so you are made whole. If you believe God created you for a purpose, you should also believe He will give you what you need to complete the good work you are called to do.

Today, allow space to listen to what God has to say to you. Many times, in prayer, the conversation is one-sided but if you are going to gain perspective on your purpose, you need to listen. It is time to be silent. Instead of listening to your regular playlist or a podcast or audiobook, turn it off and turn God on. Your goal is to listen to God, be open to what plans He has in store for you. Allow the silence to direct your thoughts and fill you with the words you need to keep the tempo and pace you need.

JOURNAL

Train today in silence and listen for God. Reflect on where He is directing you today. Ask God to give you the will and the energy to complete the good work.

Write down what you hear God saying to you.

ACTION

Do not forget to take the time to stretch before and after your exercise to help prevent injury. Plus, it is the perfect time to turn off the volume of the world and allow God to sit with you in silence.

> Level 1: spend 10-15 minutes doing a cross-training activity and take part in 10-15 minutes of a weight training activity
> Level 2: spend 20-30 minutes doing a cross-training activity and take part in 10-15 minutes of a weight training activity
> Level 3: spend 60-90 minutes doing a cross-training activity and take part in 15-20 minutes of a weight training activity

Do Not Settle

Scripture: 1 Thessalonians 5:19

> Do not quench the spirit.

REFLECTION

The scripture is concise today, 'do not quench the spirit' (1Thess 5:19). Imagine the Spirit is within you. One of the images of the Holy Spirit is fire, so think of a fire inside of you. Even go as far as imagining that all the work you have put into this challenge has been you, collecting the wood and building the framework of a fire pit. At some point, perhaps you can even identify that specific moment, the flame ignited, and the fire started. It might have been at the very beginning of the challenge or somewhere along the way, but you felt the Holy Spirit alive inside of you.

Today's scripture is supposed to encourage you to keep working toward your goal and to do your best. You have learned that on the good days when you can give 90%, God gets you the rest of the way. Then on those days when you can only give 20%, God is with you, making up for the other 80%. Do not let the fire go out on this challenge, not when you have come so far. Do not let negative thoughts creep in and make you think you need to quit because you have missed a few days of exercise or have not been able to keep up with the prayer reflections or scripture readings. Remember, on those days, God has brought you to completion.

Nowhere in the definition of disciple does it say you need to be perfect, nor does it say you even have to do everything right all the time. Instead, a disciple is a person who continuously shows up to do the work God calls them to do. One of the words used to describe a disciple is countercultural, meaning you do not go along with the crowd, instead you follow God's plan. And several times in the scripture you can read examples of how God does not do things the way the world does, and neither should a disciple. Do not settle for being mediocre.

Have you heard of the bell curve? This is a tool teachers use to grade, to find the average of what the students know. This is a valuable information for teachers but what would this look like if you used it to grade humanity on spirituality? Where would you fall on the grade scale? If God were grading on a bell curve, would you want to be average? A person who seeks to be a disciple of Jesus should work harder, should strive to get an 'A,' and not settle for anything else.

You do not want to be average; you want to be extraordinary. That is what a disciple is and that is how God sees you. Do not settle for the ordinary because God created you to be much more. Do not be caught doing average work, rather keep the spirit up and do all you can. Continue to push to be different, be countercultural, see things as God sees not as the world sees. Put more fire on the flame and continue to lean on God to see you to completion. He has begun a magnificent work in you.

JOURNAL

God is not giving out grade cards but if He were, discern your answer and why this is the grade you would get.

What grade would God give you?

Are you satisfied with your grade? What changes do you need to make?

Do you know someone who you would describe as giving an 'A' quality of effort in their discipleship? Identify the qualities they have, write them down and so you can refer to them as you cultivate them in your life.

Who do you know gets and 'A' for their effort of being a good disciple?

What qualities do they have and how can you cultivate them in your life?

ACTION

Reflect on the grade God would give you as you stretch before and after your exercise.

Level 1: participate in 20-30 minutes of a cross-training activity
Level 2: participate in 45-60 minutes of a cross-training activity
Level 3: participate in 60-90 minutes of a cross-training activity

DAY 74

Takes Courage

Scripture: Psalm 31:1-24

> Be strong, and let your heart take courage, all you
> who wait for the Lord. (Ps 31:24)

REFLECTION

It takes a lot of courage to make a commitment like what you have
with *Discipleship 5K* and following through with the physical and
spiritual practices. Over the past couple of months, you may have
tried new exercises, or reached out to someone you had previously
been afraid to talk to, or maybe even talked more openly about your
spirituality with friends and family. Courage is one of the qualities
you have exercised through this challenge.

Even the word challenge gives the impression that you will need
some courage to overcome some obstacles that will arise. And when
you talk about building your faith and standing up for what is right,
well, it can require more than an ounce of courage for most people.

The physical and spiritual exercises are designed to get you to
try new things and to push your limits. Each person will need to
draw on courage for something. There might be someone who needs
the courage to put on a pair of shorts, while another person needs
the courage to take their Bible to work. It takes courage to get out
there every day and complete the physical challenge, but you build
confidence with each step you take. You are also building courage in
your faith through the spiritual challenge and gaining confidence in
your beliefs. You have shown great courage both on the physical side
and the spiritual side. Thank you for being an example of courage.

JOURNAL

A beautiful way to pray the Bible is through the process of *Lectio Divina*. This is when you read a piece of scripture and allow words or phrases to speak to you. Today for your journal time, read Psalm 31 and choose some words or phrases that you find are a source of motivation. Read the scripture through a couple of times to really let the words marinate inside of you.

Think of the words of the scripture as macaroni noodles in a pot of boiling water and you want to wait for those first few noodles to float to the top as the macaroni is cooked. Those words that come to the top are the 3-5 words you will use over the next week to keep you motivated.

> Write down the phrases that you will use as encouragement this week.

As you read scripture and apply it to your life, you become more courageous to speak to others about God, faith, and religion because you have spent time learning about it. Talk to someone about the discipleship training and share with them how it has helped build up your courage both personally and spiritually.

Who will you talk to about *Discipleship 5K*?

ACTION

Focus on connecting to God through your mind, body, and spirit God through the exercise today.

> Level 1: practice 15-20 minutes of yoga or stretching
> and do 20-30 minutes of a cross-training activity
> Level 2: practice 20-40 minutes of yoga or stretching
> and do 30-45 minutes of a cross-training activity
> Level 3: practice 30-60 minutes of yoga or stretching
> and do 45-60 minutes of a cross-training activity

Ask Forgiveness

Scripture: Jeremiah 7:23

> But this command I gave them, "Obey my voice,
> and I will be your God, and you shall be my people;
> and walk only in the way that I command you, so
> that it may be well with you."

REFLECTION

This piece of scripture from the Old Testament is God giving reassurance to His people that He will be there for them and with them each step of the way on their journey. God wants what is best for them and for you. It is like when a parent or other caring adult asks a child to take their hand as they navigate to cross the street. God is asking you to take His hand so He may guide you. Trust in God, He has big plans for you (Jer 29:11-14).

God gave the commandments to His people, the Israelites, at a time when they were having a tough time figuring out how to honor God. So, he made it easy for them by giving them ten rules to follow. Then Jesus came and condensed them into two rules to follow; love God with all your heart, mind and soul and love your neighbor as yourself. That did not make them easier to follow, just easier to remember.

The commandments are not suggestions, rather they are for your own good just like when a parent tells their child not to touch a hot stove or play with matches. Not following the rules means there are consequences to suffer. When you break the commandments, you separate yourself from God and breaking God's Law is different than breaking the law in the world. If you break a law in the world, the consequence could be time spent in jail or a fine you must pay. When you do not live your life according to God's Commandments, you sin, and sin keeps you from being in good relationship with God and others.

As you prepare for the 5K race or as journey to the cross, one of the things you need to do to become a better disciple is to let go of or remove any unwanted and unnecessary baggage. When you carry around too much stress, worry, or sin, it can get heavy. It can weigh you mind and body down.

You have been focusing on becoming good physically and this week specifically, doing maintenance on parts of your body that may have been ignoring. When you do not give attention where attention is due, you can often do more damage by letting the problem go. Make sure there is not a physical ailment or a personal issue that you have been putting on the back burner. It is time to take care of it and get your mind clear of any distractions.

Now, there is a third part of getting yourself set up for success, it is checking in on your spirit. The best way to clean up your spirit is by doing an examination of conscious and getting rid of anything that is weighing you down emotionally. The words of today's scripture point directly at the Ten Commandments, which were given for the good of all people. So, when looking to remove behaviors or practices from your life that hurt God and hurt others, the best place to start is by making sure you are living your life in line with the commandments of God.

In the Catholic Church, there is a practice of telling your sins to a priest in the sacrament of reconciliation. This is also sometimes called confession. No matter what a person calls it, the action of telling your sin to a priest, who is a representative of God in the confessional, is only one part of the process. The other part is, after telling your sin and handing it over to God, in return you have penance to do. Penance is some combination of prayer and action that you are asked to complete.

Now going to a priest and telling him your sin only removes the sin you confess; it does not keep you from committing the sin again. If you genuinely want to stop committing the sin, the penance can help you refrain from the sinful behavior when you are tempted the next time.

Non-Catholic faiths also believe in the practice of asking for forgiveness of wrongs done. There are powerful stories of forgiveness where people forgive some pretty incredible deeds, and when this is done, the heavy load of sin is removed. The key is to ask for forgiveness for your wrongs and be open to forgiving those who have hurt you.

This is what God means when He says in the Scripture that you, "walk in the way that I command you, so that it may be well with you" (Jer 7:23). When you ask for forgiveness and forgive others, then you will be well because you are not carrying around festering hurts or negative thoughts or unhealthy feelings towards God or others.

JOURNAL

When you break a commandment, you 'dirty' your spirit which can separate you from God and others. Today your journal exercise is to do an examination of conscience, using the Ten Commandments as your guide. This will help prepare you for the race ahead, body, mind, and spirit.

> 1st Commandment: You shall have no other Gods before the Lord.
> Have you put other relationships or things such as work or other addictions before your relationship with God?

2nd Commandment: You shall not take the name of the Lord in vain.
Have you spoken of God in a negative light or cursed the name of the Lord?

3rd Commandment: You shall keep the Sabbath day holy.
Have you made each day just another day of work and obligation, and excluded God, not setting aside time to honor Him and give thanks for what you have been given?

4th Commandment: You shall honor your mother and father.
Have you shown respect, not only to your own mother and father, but to the elderly of the community?

Have you done all you can to help them maintain dignity?

5th Commandment: You shall not kill.
Have you knocked down another person with your words?

Have you tried to kill someone's reputation through gossip?

6th Commandment: You shall not commit adultery.
Have you taken part in immoral sexual acts on your own or with others?

7th Commandment: You shall not steal.
Have you been untrue in situations with money such as when filing taxes, seeking reimbursement, or keeping your timesheet?

8th Commandment: You shall not bear false witness. Have you intentionally lied about yourself or someone else to lead others to believe something that is untrue?

9th Commandment: You shall not covet your neighbor's wife.
Have you had impure thoughts of another human?

10th Commandment: You shall not covet your neighbor's goods.
Have you been jealous of another person or acted out of greed?

ACTION

Spend time before and after your walk or run stretching and doing at least 10 minutes of calisthenics.

Level 1: walk 2-3 miles as fast as you can
Level 2: run 2.5-4 miles at your peak pace
Level 3: run 4-8 miles at your peak pace

DAY 76

Nothing Easy

Scripture: Psalm 30:5

> For his anger is but for a moment; his favor is for a lifetime. Weeping may linger for the night, but joy comes with the morning.

REFLECTION

There is so much to gain as a disciple of Christ but the road to get there is rough and ragged. You might get weary and need to rest, you might stumble and fall, you might even shed a few tears but when you keep your focus on Christ as your end goal, you will succeed. If the road were easy, would it be worth it in the end?

Remember this when you are walking or running in the 5K. There might be a few potholes, or you might get tripped up or a hill might kick your butt. Do not let the obstacles get in the way of your goal. Just as you have had obstacles come up as you have been training, you persevere through and face them as they come. Trust that you are prepared to face the potholes on the path.

Today's scripture says that God has favor in you for a lifetime. He is your cheerleader and continues to be for this race and beyond. This is great news, because even if you do get tripped up along the way, it is okay. God loves you even if you do not do everything right. God is not going to hold a grudge and be mad at you, instead He is going to be proud of your effort, no matter what. There will be hard times. The scripture passage even says there will be weeping but hold on because the joy is coming. A celebration is just around the corner.

Jesus is the best example of this. Jesus was crucified and was raised from the dead to show the promise of God's love. You will suffer but when you believe in the resurrection, you believe the promise that good will prevail. Put your beliefs into actions and get out there and do this challenge to the best of your ability. When you look back on the experience, you will be in awe of what you accomplished because God was there with you every step of the way.

JOURNAL

The journal exercise for Day 75 was a doozy. Today, spend time thinking about the journal exercise from yesterday and specifically on any potentially lingering problems, issues, baggage, or sin that might still be hanging on. The practice of a daily examination of conscious is supposed to keep you focused on God and the path He has planned for you. The *Daily Examen*, is a core practice of Ignatian Spirituality and first began with Saint Ignatius of Loyola, the Catholic Saint who began the Jesuit Order of Priests. He believed a regular practice of looking back on your day, the conversations you had with others and the thoughts that consumed your mind, could guide you towards being a better disciple. This practice has been successful for many because when done daily, you can begin to see patterns in your thoughts and behaviors. It also highlights where sin is creeping in and where you get tripped up or distracted from your goals. You can also start to identify the 'God moments' you have throughout the day and more readily see God's blessings as they come. To learn more about the *Daily Examen*, go online to search the many resources on the topic.

Write down anything still holding on after yesterday's reflection.

ACTION

Spend your walk and yoga time in silence so you can listen for God's guidance.

> Level 1: take a 2–4-mile leisurely walk and practice 10-15 minutes of yoga or stretching
> Level 2: take a 3–5-mile leisurely walk or jog and practice 15-20 minutes of yoga or stretching
> Level 3: take a 5–7-mile leisurely jog and practice 20-30 minutes of yoga or stretching

All In

Scripture: Mark 8:34-38

> He called the crowd with is disciples, and said to them, 'If any of you want to become my followers, let them deny themselves and take up their cross and follow me.' (Mark 8:34)

REFLECTION

The scripture says if you lose your life for the sake of Jesus, or for the sake of the Gospel, you have gained eternal life. God is promising a big reward but in return, you must do some challenging work. It is not always easy to stand up for what is right or even to do the right thing all the time. When you began this challenge, what was the primary motivation? Most likely it was to work toward having a better relationship with God and maybe to be able to improve your physical health. Either way it was to make some kind of improvement in your life and by now the change in you physically and spiritually is evident. Maybe not to everyone who sees you each day, but you know you are different.

All the work you did to overcome the obstacles involved in some of the physical challenges and even a few of the spiritual challenges may have taken a toll on you. So, when you complete the work, you may be so overjoyed and tempted to take on all the glory for your accomplishments. However, if you have learned anything and what this scripture is reminding you, is that you do all things for the glory of God. Yes, you can be proud of all the good that has occurred and of course a better relationship with God is definitely worth celebrating. But at the end of the day, this challenge is about doing what it takes to be a better disciple and that means through your words and actions. In the end, you shine God's light brighter.

Disney had a series of movies called, *High School Musical.* One of the songs was titled, "In It to Win It," which is sung by a character who, after facing some adversity, decides he is going to go after his goal. This is the theme song for you at this point in the challenge. The commitment you made when you began the journey of *Discipleship 5K* was a big one and along the way you have made some even bigger sacrifices. You have come so far on this journey both physically and spiritually. The fact you are still doing the work must mean you are all in, you are in it to win it too.

JOURNAL

Make a list of eleven things you have enjoyed most about the past eleven weeks. It might be something that brought you joy, it might be a goal you met, or it may be a new relationship or past relationship that has been reconciled. Write down these things and if you need inspiration or reminders, look back on your journal entries to pick out your top ten, uh, eleven list.

> Make note of eleven things that you have enjoyed over the past eleven weeks of *Discipleship 5K.*

ACTION

Choose your favorite exercise routine to do today. If there is yoga or cross-training program you enjoy, pick those but if your favorite exercise routine is something else, do that instead.

> Level 1: spend 15-20 minutes practicing yoga or stretching and 30-45 minutes taking part in a cross-training activity
> Level 2: spend 20-30 minutes practicing yoga or stretching and 45-60 minutes taking part in a cross-training activity
> Level 3: spend 30-60 minutes practicing yoga or stretching and 60-90 minutes taking part in a cross-training activity

WEEK ELEVEN OVERVIEW

Write down any thoughts, words of encouragement, ideas for growth or measurements of progress you have from this week from your physical and spiritual training.

WEEK TWELVE
The Race is Only Beginning

You can see the finish line! Remember you got this far due to a team effort, you, and God. Each day this week the scripture will give you small nugget of wisdom to help you complete the task at hand. Additionally, look at these words from Sirach 3:17-24.

> My child, perform your tasks with humility, then you will be loved by those whom God accepts. The greater you are, the more you must humble yourself, so you will find favor in the sight of the Lord. For great is the might of the Lord, bur by the humble he is glorified. Neither seek what is too difficult for you nor investigate what is beyond your power. Reflect upon what you have been commanded for what is hidden is not your concern. Do not meddle in matters that are beyond you, for more than you can understand has been shown you. For their conceit has led many astray, and wrong opinion has impaired their judgement.

Scripture offers so much and this week, make time to reflect on each verse and find encouragement and wisdom in God's words. If moved to do so, study these verses from Sirach and look for what each line is saying to you, allow this to be your motivation to finish this race and move onto whatever God has planned for you next. The race is only beginning of what you can accomplish.

DAY 78
Have Faith
Scripture: Acts 27:21-25

> So, keep up your courage, men, for I have faith in God
> that it will be exactly as I have been told. (Acts 27:25)

REFLECTION

Imagine you are in the boat with Saint Paul and have been for the past eleven weeks. There is little to do in the boat except to allow faith to dwindle away but Saint Paul has a dream that God has come to him and has promised they will all see this journey through to the end. Over the past several weeks, there might have been times when it felt the activities were monotonous, like you were doing the same thing or reading the same words over and over. You may have been so focused on your goal and the tasks at hand that you forgot there was a world around you. Whatever the case, the vision Saint Paul had, and the words of God are here for you to gain insight, strength, and purpose.

You are one week from completing a challenging thing, do not get caught up in what you should have done better or could have done more, rather concentrate on what you have done, and will do. Turn your thinking around. Like the men in the boat, if you allow, your mind will take over and send you down a slippery slope of hopelessness and despair. Remember, God does not throw pity parties, so put on those running shoes and get out there to do your physical training. Also open that Bible and read the scripture to build on your spiritual life to gain the confidence you need to succeed.

The training in *Discipleship 5K* is not about preparing for a specific for an event, rather it is training for life. You have worked hard both physically and spiritually, but you have not maxed out. Once you have completed the exercises in *Discipleship 5K*, you need to decide how you will maintain physically and spiritually the work God has begun in you.

If you were motivated to do the physical exercise because there was a race to complete, then sign up for another race. If not, figure out what did motivate you to move your body each day and replicate it. Perhaps the motivating factor was that you had found a group of friends to work out with and if you stop doing the exercise then you will miss the camaraderie and support of others. You do not need to stop just because you are at the end of this particular training. Keep going, hold yourself accountable to set and meet physical goals each day, week, or month. Discipleship training never stops.

Additionally, there are several ways you can continue to grow and build the relationship you have more deeply developed with God, Jesus, and the Holy Spirit. Find a Bible study or begin one. Seek ways you can volunteer in your community. Make a point to do random acts of kindness each day. The most important piece to all of this is to remain close to God, continue to speak to Him and listen.

As you complete this week, it is okay to be thinking about the answer to the 'what is next' question. Taking a few moments to consider how you might use your gifts in the future could help you forget about what could have been and keep you focused on what will be. There are no regrets when you are mindful and living in the present. Instead of looking at past mistakes or regrets or thinking about being stuck in a boat without the prospect of getting out, remain strong in the faith. Take courage in the knowledge that God is there and will be with you through whatever is ahead. God has been here all along.

JOURNAL

Today, reflect on the people, places and things that make you feel grounded and connected. The scripture is a good reminder to stay strong and courageous and have faith.

> Draw a picture of an anchor for a ship and write in the people in your life who keep you anchored in your relationship with God. Then define what it means to you to be anchored.

ACTION

Stretching and strengthening your muscles help you build endurance so be sure you are spending 5-10 minutes before and after your exercise.

> Level 1: walk 2-3 miles as fast as you can and do 5 minutes of calisthenics
> Level 2: run 2.5-4 miles at your peak pace and do 10 minutes of calisthenics
> Level 3: run 4-8 miles at your peak pace and do 10 minutes of calisthenics

Stay Connected

Scripture: Genesis 28:10-22

> Then Jacob made a vow, saying, 'If God will be
> with me, and will keep me in this way that I go,
> and will give me bread to eat and clothing to wear.'
> (Gen 28:20)

REFLECTION

Over the past twelve weeks you have spent each day in the Word,
reading scripture and reflecting on it. Surely you have come to know
Jesus more deeply though the readings and the reflections. You have
learned or been affirmed that God is with you always, Jesus lives
within you and the Spirit is all around you. This practice of time
spent in the Word of God daily does not have to stop once you have
completed the training. Discipleship training never ends, and you
need to continue to work on your relationship with God just as you
work on your family and friend relationships. You must continue to
reach out to God, seeking him in your thoughts and your actions.

JOURNAL

Pick a symbol, image, or trinket to use as a reminder to stay
connected to scripture once the challenge is over. Consider using a
rock like Jacob did or a prayer card or what many followers use as
their reminder, the cross.

What will you use as your symbol, image, or trinket to remind you to stay connected to scripture?

On Day 35 you wrote down several ways you could get involved in something that would help keep you connected to the good habits you have created through the work in *Discipleship 5K*. Add to these ideas by thinking of ways you could use the tools of connection such as reaching out to someone via a phone call, Facetime or Zoom. Consider how you might text positive words or scripture to a different friend or family member each day or how you might use encouraging words to motivate one another to get up and move your bodies for at least 30 minutes each day. You could use social media platforms such as Facebook, Instagram, Snapchat, Twitter, TikTok or wherever you and your friends spend time together.

It is important to find ways to encourage one another and show support, especially when it comes to making choices about physical and spiritual health and overall welfare. Of course, connecting in person is even better. It is always fun to meet friends at a coffee shop or for happy hour to exchange stories of success and brainstorm ideas on how to face challenges. Create a plan. Choose one idea and do it each day or put a reminder on your phone or in your calendar to do one of these things or to schedule to do one of these things daily, weekly, or monthly. You were given the task to think about it and now it is time to put a concrete plan in place.

How can you use your phone to connect more deeply to someone?

How can you use text to connect to others more regularly?

How can you use your favorite social media platform to connect to friends and family?

How can you connect to others in person more regularly?

What are things you can do daily to deepen my relationships?

What are things you can do weekly to connect to others?

What are things you can do monthly to encourage others?

ACTION

Think of ways you can connect with others through your exercise time and prayer time.

> Level 1: practice yoga or stretching for 15-20 minutes and spend 20-30 minutes taking part in a cross-training activity
>
> Level 2: practice yoga or stretching for 20-40 minutes and spend 30-45 minutes taking part in a cross-training activity
>
> Level 3: practice yoga or stretching for 30-60 minutes and spend 45-60 minutes taking part in a cross-training activity

Holy Living

Scripture: 1 Peter 1:13-25

> Like obedient children, do not be conformed to the
> desires that you formerly had in ignorance. Instead,
> as he who called you is holy, be holy yourselves in
> all your conduct; for it is written, "You shall be holy,
> for I am holy." (1 Pet 1:14-16)

REFLECTION

Read the entire passage, not just what is written here. There is so
much more to read, and you need time to allow it to sink in. The
words here though, you have heard them before along this journey;
not just once, but twice. Remember, it comes from the book of
Leviticus, where in chapter 19 you read about all the things you
should do so you can be holy and then chapter 20 lists all the things
that would defile you.

The fact Saint Peter is the one speaking in this passage is a
reminder that everyone can be holy. So often in the Gospel stories it
is Peter who is questioning Jesus and making a fool of himself. Peter,
or Simon as he was known prior to Jesus calling him to be one of
the first disciples. Peter is the one who stepped out of the boat and
sank when he took his eyes off Jesus (Matt 14:29). Peter suggested
they build three tents on the mountain top after the Transfiguration
experience. He did not understand that they were being called to
action, and it was not time to recline (Matt 17:4). He is the one to
questioned Jesus about why Jesus did not stand up and fight against
the Sadducees and Pharisees who were trying to trap him into doing
or saying something that could get him arrested (Matt 16:23). And

of course, Peter is the one who denied even knowing Jesus the night of the crucifixion (Matt 26:69-75).

However, Peter did many things right. He rarely let Jesus out of his sight, and when Jesus asked who Peter believed He was, Peter knew Jesus was the Son of God (Luke 9:18-20). Peter gave up his family and his job to follow Jesus (Luke 5:1-11) and because of the sacrifice, Jesus crowned him with the honor of being the first Pope of the Catholic Church (Matt 16:18).

Jesus knew Peter was obedient to the faith and to Him, even though he had messed up and did not always do what was right. Peter is an excellent example of a disciple. He learned by making mistakes, but he stuck with it because he knew it was worth doing. In the end, follow these five steps and you are sure to get it right too.

1. Discipline yourself
2. Set your hope in Christ
3. Follow God's Law
4. Seek truth in all things
5. Spread the Good News

JOURNAL

A call to holy living, this is what being a disciple is about. These past weeks you have worked hard to build, strengthen, and maintain a relationship with God, and this will not end as long as you continue to put in the work. Remember anything worth having requires work.

> How will you live out the Gospel message of serving God and others?

How will you seek the wisdom of the scriptures?

How will you exercise self-discipline physically and spiritually?

How will you build endurance physically and spiritually?

How will you keep courage to speak the truth?

ACTION

Take a few minutes to stretch before and after your exercise. When you practice your breathing, imagine breathing in the things that are holy and breathing out the things that are not holy.

Level 1: walk 1.5-3 miles at a moderate pace
Level 2: jog 2-4 miles at a moderate pace
Level 3: run 4-8 miles at a moderate pace

DAY 81

Keep Your Promise

Scripture: Numbers 30:2

> When a man makes a vow to the Lord or swears an oath to bind himself by a pledge, he shall not break his word; he shall do according to all that proceeds out of his mouth.

REFLECTION

There is a difference between when God makes a promise and others make a promise because God's word is always truth. This cannot be said for human beings. From the beginning of creation, Adam and Eve set the course for human nature to be a sinful nature. When another person says they promise something, it is not guaranteed like when God promises.

It is this truth that makes it a crime to tell a lie when under oath in a court of law. There is a long history of human beings not being truthful or honest. However, there is an entire book called the Bible full of evidence of God fulfilling his promises. It is especially shown when God sacrifices his own son, Jesus. Every Christian person knows that Jesus died on the cross to forgive sins and when He rose from the dead, it was a sign to all that whoever believes in God will rise with Jesus on the last day.

A little more than twelve weeks ago, you made a promise to God and to yourself to begin the journey of *Discipleship 5K*. And soon the words of Saint Paul to the Philippians will be true of you too when he said, "I am confident of this, that the one who began a good work among you will bring it to completion" (Phil 1:6). God has been there with you each step of the way and will continue to be with you once the challenge is over.

However, the journey to the cross for a disciple is never over, not until you reach the final destination, heaven. Today it is time to ask the question, 'how will you continue to work on your physical and spiritual health now that you are in the habit of doing so?' You have several options, some of which you could look back in your journal and see the seeds God planted along the way.

Physically, there might be some activities that you want to continue, especially if you have a walking buddy or are taking a class at a fitness center. As for spiritually, you have brainstormed ways to volunteer, and perhaps you are doing this already. Although the general instructions and guidelines put forth in *Discipleship 5K* have been completed, it does not mean the end of you giving your time, talent and treasure to an organization or business where you can continue to have influence. You may decide to sign up for a retreat at a local retreat center on a weekend or schedule an hour or two each week to brown bag your lunch and spend your lunch hour reading scripture or a book on spirituality.

The possibilities are endless. You just need to decide what you will do to continue to make the world a better place with your words and your actions. You are a new creation and have come too far to go back to your old habits. Get out there and complete the work that was started in you; you are not done yet.

JOURNAL

Make a vow, take an oath, and promise yourself and God to continue your discipleship training to stay strong and grow in faith. Write it here but also make a note of it to put somewhere you will see it every day like on your refrigerator or make it the screensaver on your computer or phone. You definitely want to do your best to keep your promise to God.

What is your vow, oath or promise?

ACTION

It is still important to stretch before and after you exercise, do not skip it. Make a promise to yourself that you will remember to stretch.

>Level 1: participate in 20-30 minutes of a cross-training activity
>Level 2- participate in 45-60 minutes of a cross-training activity
>Level 3- participate in 60-90 minutes of a cross-training activity

Blood - Sweat - Tears

Scripture: 2 Timothy 1:13-14

> Hold to the standard of sound teaching that you have heard from me, in the faith and love that are in Jesus. Guard the good treasure entrusted to you, with the help of the Holy Spirit living in us.

REFLECTION

You have endured 82 days of scripture, prayer, and reflection. You have also worked out your body and pushed it to new limits. You have sweat, you have suffered, you have applied the icy hot to your sore muscles, evidence you have worked hard. You have also sacrificed time, spent money, and had your share of hardships achieving the daily challenges in the reflections and actions. You have spent the past twelve weeks forming yourself into a better disciple who is not afraid to tell others what you have endured to get to this point in the training.

Throughout the challenge there have been standards of a disciple you have been held up to and through the challenge you have done the work to meet them. The scripture says you need continue to hold true and live your life according to these standards. And by now you should know you will not be doing it alone, for like Jesus, when He left the disciples for good, He left for them the Holy Spirit to remain with them. The Holy Spirit is here with you too.

Yes, there were challenging times over the past twelve weeks but those should not be all you see when you look back. You need to remember all you have learned and how strong you have become both physically and spiritually. These are the things that can push you forward into the next steps for you.

In life you can guarantee there will be some blood, sweat and tears lost but God responds with faith, hope and love to mend, repair and renew whatever is broken. God's goodness and glory will wash away whatever stands in your way of completing the mission for which you were created. Keep going, God has great plans for you! (Jer 29:11-14)

JOURNAL

Spend time thinking of five things that you will carry with you onto your next challenge. Identify those things that you have developed or strengthened that will give you success in keeping the momentum you have begun to be a better version of yourself. Then write down the five things, being extremely specific, about how participation in *Discipleship 5K* has helped you become a better disciple and how you will carry that into the future.

> Name five things you will carry with you to your next challenge.

> Name five things you learned to help you continue to become a better disciple in the future.

ACTION

Push yourself to work up a really good sweat during your exercise session.

> Level 1: spend 15-20 minutes practicing yoga or stretching and 30-45 minutes taking part in a cross-training activity
>
> Level 2: spend 20-30 minutes practicing yoga or stretching and 45-60 minutes taking part in a cross-training activity
>
> Level 3: spend 30-60 minutes practicing yoga or stretching and 60-90 minutes taking part in a cross-training activity

Overcome the Odds

Scripture: 1 Corinthians 9:24-27

Run in such a way that you may win it. (1 Cor 9:24b)

REFLECTION

In an actual race, there is only one person who can cross the finish line first but that does not mean they are the only winner. There are some who run the race because they want to be a part of something or to stand up for a cause and they are winners too. Some push themselves to get a better time and strive to reach a personal best and they are winners as well.

For you, the completion of the twelve-week journey of the *Discipleship 5K* training gives you a gold medal. You have put in the work, made sacrifices, and learned a little self-discipline. To God, everyone wins the race as long as you enter it. But as a disciple you do not just want to enter, instead you want to give it your all to reach your goal. Look to examples in scripture and in the world of people who have overcome huge obstacles to follow the path before them.

There are several examples of people who overcome extraordinary odds to fulfill their purpose. A couple of examples include, Bethany Dillon, who persevered to achieve her dream of being a professional surfer even after losing her arm in a shark attack. And Michael Jordan, legendary basketball player who was not considered good enough to make his high school team but went on to play in the NBA, notably taking the sport to a whole new level. These and many others have goals and work hard to achieve their goals, but it takes time, persistence, and focus. You need to continue to get out there every day and spend time getting stronger physically and mentally, which is like what you have done in your *Discipleship 5K* training.

JOURNAL

Find others who have overcome hard things while working towards achieving a goal. It can be a story of someone who is known to many, like Bethany Dillon or Michael Jordan, or it can be someone who has inspired you with how they tackled a challenging thing. Consider looking up William Kyle Carpenter, Amberley Snyder or search the internet for other examples of people who persevere to achieve a personal goal. You might know someone personally who has overcome great odds to fulfill a purpose. Whomever you choose and wherever you find inspiration, today, as you finish Day 83 of an 84-day challenge, you are in their company.

> Write the name of a person whose story has made an impact on your life because of the way they overcame an obstacle.

> What about their story inspires you or what lesson does it teach you?

Can you think of more than one?
Write the name of a person whose story has made an impact on your life because of the way they overcame an obstacle.

What about their story inspires you or what lesson does it teach you?

ACTION

Take a day of rest if you think it is needed.

Level 1: take a 2–4-mile leisurely walk and spend 10-15 minutes doing yoga or stretching
Level 2: take a 3–5-mile leisurely walk or jog and spend 15-20 minutes doing yoga or stretching
Level 3: take a 5–7-mile leisurely jog and spend 20-30 minutes doing yoga or stretching

DAY 84

Blessed Are You

Scripture: James 1:2-18

> Blessed is anyone who endures temptation. Such one has stood the test and will receive the crown of life that the Lord has promised to those who love him. (Jas 1:12)

REFLECTION

You have made some great strides in your physical and spiritual journey. It is time to stop and reflect on where you have been and consider the possibilities of where you will go next. Today, make time to be still and quiet as you read the reflection. It is a guided meditation. It is not something you simply read through and ponder on later, rather it is something you need to read slowly, one line at a time. It can be a really powerful exercise and something you might find value in doing once or twice a year to help you remain connected to God and focused on your discipleship.

Before you begin:
Find a quiet spot in your home or even outside where you can sit comfortably.

When you are settled, practice your breathing exercises to relax your body and clear your mind.

Begin to slowly read each sentence aloud so the words can surround your body.

Imagine yourself taking a walk on your favorite path. Take a deep breathe in as you smell the fresh air and feel a gentle breeze touch your skin.

Notice how the wind moves the leaves in the trees making the sunlight shimmer and dance in the shadows.

As you walk, you begin to notice symbols and images that bring back memories from your life.

You see a child riding a bike like the one you rode as a child.

And ahead you see a stretch of road that reminds you of a vacation you took.

With each step, you realize the path you are on is a representation of your life.

You continue to see things that highlight good times and bad times.

Your mind is on overload as you catch glimpses of obstacles you have faced, temptations you have overcome and some that still plague you.

Your achievements, goals you have reached, things you are proud of rush to the forefront of your mind. And as you walk, you are surprised at how much you have accomplished so far in your life.

You stop for a moment to catch your breath and take in the flood of memories.

Put a name to what you are feeling.

Is it pride or satisfaction?

Is it regret or sorrow?

Identify the feeling.

Before you begin to walk again, look back on the path where you have already been.

As you look behind you, all the images and memories blend together in a cloud as though they are being protected and held for you to revisit.

When you are ready, you turn around to resume walking forward.

You see a figure of a person coming towards you.

It is difficult to see them as they are a good distance away.

As you walk towards each other, you recognize the figure.

It is Jesus.

When you realize it is Jesus coming, what do you feel?

Are you happy or excited?

Are you embarrassed or nervous?

When you finally approach each other, Jesus reaches out to embrace you in a hug.

You stand there holding each other while Jesus whispers, "it is good to see you here."

What is your response to Jesus?

He asks if you would like to sit with him for a while.

You agree and sit down together on a bench.

Jesus asks you how you are doing.

What is your response?

You sit together for a while talking about your life, the highs, and the lows.

You tell Jesus about the things you have learned through these experiences, and you ask Him questions.

What are the questions you ask Jesus?

Jesus thanks you for sharing your memories with Him.

You stand and Jesus reaches out to give you another hug.

He tells you He is proud of you for getting this far on your journey.

Jesus asks if He can continue walking the path with you.

You and Jesus get up and start walking together.

As you begin walking again, you feel different, you feel lighter, but you also feel full.

You realize that with Jesus, you feel more confident and capable of accomplishing whatever you need to and know with Him by your side, you can overcome anything that comes your way.

Jesus' presence with you right now solidifies that He has been there all along.

He has provided you opportunities in your life to grow into deeper relationship with Him.

And you know on the road ahead, Jesus will continue to walk with you, step by step.

JOURNAL

The scripture says God will reward you for the work you have done. This means you get to celebrate today the completion of your *Discipleship 5K* journey, but it is not the end of the road for you. God has big plans for you, bigger than everything you have done to this point. Your commitment, dedication, and perseverance to complete this challenge shows you are made for more and you have proven that by making it all the way to today. Reflect on this journey of preparing yourself physically and spiritually for the 5K.

What is the biggest change in you physically?

What is the biggest change in you spiritually?

What are you most looking forward to in the future physically?

What are you most looking forward to in the future spiritually?

Lastly, what would you say to someone who has never heard of the *Discipleship 5K*?

ACTION

Whether you have plans to run an actual race or simply the race of life, remember the end goal is to reach the cross, and Jesus is there with you every step of the way. Keep up the good work!

ADDITIONAL RESOURCES

THE DISCIPLESHIP 5K COMMUNITY

Disciples are called to fulfill a mission, they have purpose. You are a disciple and thus are one of many called by God. In the Gospel of Luke, Jesus tells the disciples before they are sent that, "the harvest is plentiful, but the laborers are few; therefore ask the Lord of the harvest to send out laborers to his harvest" (Luke 10:2). The *Discipleship 5K* Community is where you will find other disciples laboring to fulfill the mission for which they have been called.

There are a couple of ways you can get connected to the *Discipleship 5K* Community. The best way is to find *Making Scripture Relevant* on Facebook, Instagram, and YouTube. Each of these social media platforms offer something different to support and motivate you along the journey.

The Facebook page has a specific *Discipleship 5K* Community, a group of disciples in training, where you can ask questions, share your successes, and offer encouragement to others. The Instagram page offers daily inspirational images based on scripture, with prayers and reflections. On the YouTube channel, you will find 3–5-minute videos for each day of *Discipleship 5K* where the Author shares insights on the daily scripture and reflection, giving additional resources and encouraging you along the way.

ABOUT THE AUTHOR

Heather Neds has been a ministry leader for over 20 years, sharing the gospel message. Her personal passion and dedication to nurturing the mind, body, spirit relationship is something she has worked to develop in her own life since she was in middle school. She feels called to help people have an intimate relationship with God and believes it starts in the scriptures. In her personal and professional life, she has helped middle school and high school teens, as well as countless adults cultivate and deepen their faith through prayer, reflection, and retreat experiences.

She is self-taught in topics of diet, exercise, and healthy lifestyles; turning to physical activity to manage stress and a positive body image. It was when she began putting in more time and effort into developing her faith that she found the disciplines to be the same as the disciplines of making healthy choices. In a world where there are not enough hours in the day to complete the tasks you would like; Heather provides an effective way to double down and use exercise time as prayer time and vice versa.

Heather Neds leads a Scripture study at Keeler Women's Center, a ministry of the Benedictine Sisters in Atchison KS. She has authored articles for Celebration Publication and Catholic Fam Magazine and worked as a youth minister for 15 years in the Diocese of Kansas City-St. Joseph. Her story is featured in Voyage Austin Magazine, an online platform promoting entrepreneurs. Her passion for scripture led to the development of the blog *Making Scripture Relevant*, where she shares life/faith stories on the website and daily reflections and prayers on social media.

She lives near Austin, Texas with her husband where they spend time enjoying the simple things in life. Heather is an off-road enthusiast whether on foot, her mountain bike or in her Jeep, she is never without a smile when she is out on the trails or talking about Jesus.

Discipleship 5K: A Physical and Spiritual Journey to the Cross is her first book but is a project she has been sculpting her whole life. Heather is a teacher and spiritual leader at heart. Look for a series of books with prayers and journal questions to be used alone or as a guide for groups wanting to spend time reflecting on the scriptures and where God is moving in their lives. Connect with her on social media platforms @makingscripturerelevant for daily inspiration, prayers, and reflections as well as resources for *Discipleship 5K*.

Printed in the United States
by Baker & Taylor Publisher Services